The Essential Heart Book for Women

Also by Morris Notelovitz, M.D., Ph.D., and Diana Tonnessen

Stand Tall! The Informed Woman's Guide to
  Preventing Osteoporosis (also with Marsha Ware, M.D.)
Menopause and Midlife Health
Estrogen: Yes or No?

The Essential Heart Book for Women

MORRIS NOTELOVITZ, M.D., Ph.D.,
and
DIANA TONNESSEN

Illustrations and tables by Nikki Stewart

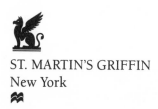

ST. MARTIN'S GRIFFIN
New York

Permissions Acknowledgments can be found on page 305.

Library of Congress Cataloging-in-Publication Data

Notelovitz, Morris.
    The essential heart book for women / Morris Notelovitz and Diana Tonnessen ; illustrations by Nikki Stewart.—1st ed.
        p. cm.
    Includes bibliographical references and index.
    ISBN 0-312-15524-7
        1. Cardiovascular system—Diseases.   2. Women—Diseases.   3. Cardiovascular system—Diseases—Sex factors.   I. Tonnessen, Diana.   II. Title.
    RC669.N68   1996
    616.1'0082—dc20   95-41703
                                                                                                    CIP

First St. Martin's Griffin Edition: June 1997

10 9 8 7 6 5 4 3 2 1

Contents

PREFACE   ix

INTRODUCTION   "But My Cholesterol Is 'Normal,' " and Other   1
Myths

PART I   *What Is Cardiovascular Disease?*

CHAPTER 1   The Healthy Heart   13

CHAPTER 2   How Men and Women Are Different   25

PART II   *Coronary Artery Disease*

CHAPTER 3   How Coronary Artery Disease Develops   33

CHAPTER 4   Are You at Risk?   48

CHAPTER 5   Common Screening and Diagnostic Tests   64

CHAPTER 6   A Prudent Diet for the Prevention of   80
Coronary Artery Disease

CHAPTER 7   Exercising Your Option for a Healthier Heart   117

CHAPTER 8   Other Ways to Reduce Your Risk   133

CHAPTER 9   Should You Take Estrogen?   146

CHAPTER 10   Drugs Used to Prevent Coronary Artery   175
Disease

CHAPTER 11   If You Already Have Coronary Artery Disease   181

CHAPTER 12   If You Have a Heart Attack   202

PART III   *Other Forms of Cardiovascular Disease*

CHAPTER 13   Hypertension   211

CHAPTER 14   Stroke   226

CHAPTER 15   Other Cardiovascular Conditions   243

EPILOGUE   255
RESOURCES AND SUPPORT   256
GLOSSARY   261
SELECTED BIBLIOGRAPHY   269
APPENDIX   283
INDEX   297

PREFACE

THE WORD IS OUT: Heart disease is no longer a "man's problem"; it is increasingly being recognized as a major health threat to women, too. Indeed, heart disease is the most common cause of death in women, accounting for more deaths than breast, ovarian, and endometrial cancer combined.

Over the past several years, some disturbing gender differences have come to light regarding the development and treatment of heart disease. If you happen to be one of the half million women who develop heart trouble each year, the prognosis is not as good for you as it is for a man. For example, women who undergo invasive procedures to restore blood flow to the heart, such as angioplasty and coronary bypass surgery, experience more complications than men. And the procedures don't relieve chest pain as effectively in women as in men. Even more disturbing is the fact that heart attacks are more likely to be fatal for women than for men. So in spite of the incredible advances made in the treatment of heart disease over the past twenty years, women who develop heart problems are at a distinct disadvantage.

Clearly, for women, prevention is the key. It makes infinitely more sense to adopt a sensible diet, keep physically active, and make other necessary lifestyle modifications to reduce your risk before trouble begins than to do little more than hope that you don't develop heart problems, or to take your chances on invasive treatments that—at the present time, at least—are more risky and less effective in women than they are in men.

Where does the gynecologist fit into the picture? At the very beginning: before heart trouble develops. Gynecologists are in a unique position to help women prevent heart disease, for a number of reasons. First, if you're like most women, your gynecologist has become your primary care provider, the physician you see most regularly, and the one you turn to first when health problems arise. Second, your menopause is a turning point in terms of your risk of developing heart disease. After menopause, when estrogen levels fall, you become more vulnerable to heart problems. The menopausal years are a time when you would normally visit your gynecologist for guidance through this transition. That guidance should naturally include a program to help you prevent one of the most serious long-term complications of your menopause: heart disease. Third, your gynecologist is familiar with and comfortable prescribing estrogen, a drug that is increasingly being regarded as a powerful weapon in the fight against heart disease in women.

Here at the Women's Medical and Diagnostic Center in Gainesville, Florida. One of the first clinics in the country to cater exclusively to the health needs of women in the middle and later years—we naturally took an interest in heart disease as one of the more serious long-term complications of menopause. A main focus of our research has been to investigate the effects of one of the most widely prescribed drugs today—estrogen—on a woman's risk of cardiovascular disease. For example, we are one of a growing number of researchers to demonstrate the safety of the newer, low-dose oral contraceptives in older premenopausal women. In addition, we have conducted extensive research on the effects of various postmenopausal estrogen preparations (pills, patches, pellets) on such cardiovascular risk factors as cholesterol, insulin, glucose tolerance, blood coagulants (substances that promote the development of blood clots), and blood pressure.

We are also helping to address one of the more pressing questions facing postmenopausal women today: whether taking progestogen (a synthetic form of the reproductive hormone progesterone) along with estrogen to protect against uterine cancer will cancel out the protective effect that estrogen has on the heart and blood vessels.

In addition, we have investigated the selective use of androgens—better known as the "male" reproductive hormone testosterone. Androgens are sometimes prescribed along with estrogen for the relief of menopausal symptoms. Although the use of oral androgens can lower levels of protective high-density lipoproteins (HDL cholesterol), which is associated with an increased risk of heart disease in women, non-oral forms of androgens don't have this effect and may safely be used by postmenopausal women.

Our research hasn't been limited to the effects of hormones on a woman's risk of heart disease. We also recognized the importance of regular moderate exercise in maintaining cardiovascular health in the middle and later years. To that end, we have conducted studies on the effects of exercise on various risk factors for heart disease in women, such as blood lipids (fat and cholesterol), blood pressure, insulin, and weight. We also developed a modified version of the graded exercise stress test especially for women in midlife.

Perhaps most important of all, we have put our study findings into practice—the practice of medicine, that is. At our clinic, we routinely help women determine their cardiovascular risk, including blood-cholesterol and selective exercise testing. We then help ease women at risk into a rigorous program of prevention, one that includes a sensible, low-fat diet, regular moderate exercise and, when necessary, medication, including estrogen.

The program of prevention, described in the pages that follow, has helped numerous women reduce their risk of heart disease. Why not put it to work for you now?

"But My Cholesterol Is 'Normal,'" and Other Myths

DEBORAH WAS NOT TAKEN IN by the biggest myth about women and heart disease—that it couldn't happen to her. She had read in a magazine article that being fifty-five years old and past menopause put her at increased risk of developing heart disease. She had also read that knowing her cholesterol level could help determine just how at-risk she was. So she had her total cholesterol level tested with a finger-prick test at a health fair.

When Deborah learned the results, she breathed a sigh of relief. Her cholesterol level was in the "desirable" range, putting her at a low risk of having a heart attack. Not bad, she thought to herself. At least she didn't have to worry about heart disease.

Seven months later, however, Deborah developed chest pain. To her surprise, a diagnostic workup revealed that one of her coronary arteries was 75 percent occluded.

Deborah was somewhat more informed than the average woman. She knew enough to have her cholesterol tested to see if she was at risk of developing heart disease. Unfortunately, she didn't have enough information to evaluate her risk properly. And like so many women today, she fell victim to the numerous fictions and half-truths about women and heart disease. Unfortunately, this kind of misinformation can keep you from taking the steps needed to prevent cardiovascular problems or from getting the necessary medical attention should you happen to develop heart trouble. Do you recognize any of the following myths?

MYTH: Cardiovascular disease is a "man's illness."
FACT: This is the most widespread and dangerous myth of all because it permits women and their doctors to deny that a problem even exists. Make no mistake: while men tend to develop heart and blood vessel problems at an earlier age than women, *cardiovascular disease is the leading cause of death of both men and women in America today.* And while most women enjoy a kind of built-in biological protection against heart disease during their reproductive years, that protection begins to fade after menopause, when levels of the reproductive hormone estrogen plummet (see Table 1). After age sixty, the number of men and women who die of cardiovascular disease is the same: one in four.

MYTH: Cancer is a much more serious health threat to women than heart attacks.
FACT: Cancer is a real threat to women, but cardiovascular disease is an even greater one. Consider these statistics:

- Every year, twice as many women die of cardiovascular disease than of cancer. According to the American Heart Association, all cardiovascular diseases combined claim the lives of more than 478,000 women annually, compared with 237,000 women for all forms of cancer.
- Breast cancer claims the lives of about 43,300, women each year. But coronary artery disease, the most common form of cardiovascular disease, kills 250,000 women every year—six times more women than are killed by breast cancer.

Most women know how to examine their breasts to detect early signs of breast cancer. Yet how many women have had a lipid profile during the last five years to help determine their risk of developing heart disease?

MYTH: Only older women have to worry about heart disease.
FACT: More than one-sixth of all people killed by cardiovascular disease are under the age of sixty-five. One in seven women between the ages of forty-five and sixty-four has had some form of heart disease or stroke.

For reasons that are not yet clear, African-American women are more vulnerable than Caucasian women. Moreover, some women—those with diabetes and those with a strong family history of premature heart disease, for example—never benefit from the protection that gender provides most

TABLE 1 — Death Rates From Coronary Heart Disease:
A Comparison of Men and Women

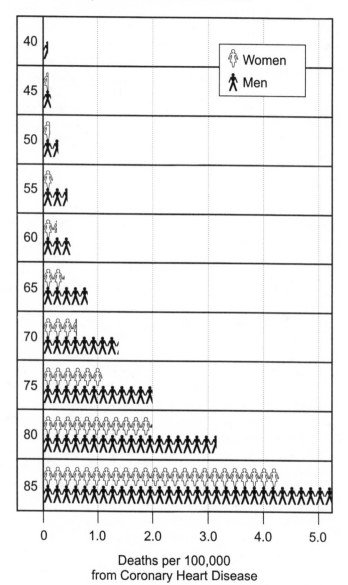

Deaths per 100,000
from Coronary Heart Disease

healthy women. These women are just as vulnerable to cardiovascular disease as are men, and at just as early an age.

Lois's story is a case in point. Her mother, her sister and her two brothers had all developed cardiovascular problems, including heart disease, high blood pressure, and stroke, which meant that Lois was at risk, too. Then Lois had a premature menopause at age thirty-two, which further increased her risk. Although she began taking postmenopausal hormones, known to confer protection against heart disease in postmenopausal women, she stopped using them after only a few months. To add insult to injury, she smoked half a pack of cigarettes a day. (Cigarette smoking is a major risk factor for heart disease.) When she was forty, Lois began having chest pains. The diagnosis: obstruction of three of her coronary arteries, requiring bypass surgery. Lois's strong family history of heart disease, combined with a premature menopause and cigarette smoking, all worked to make her vulnerable to heart disease at a much earlier age than the average woman.

Even young, healthy women in their reproductive years have good reason to be concerned about heart disease. There's strong evidence to suggest that the disease process leading to coronary artery disease begins early in life—even as early as adolescence. Recent studies involving autopsies of men and women who died of causes unrelated to cardiovascular disease have found evidence of the fatty streaks that eventually develop into artery-narrowing plaques in girls as young as age fifteen! So in terms of prevention, it's never too early to take steps to protect yourself.

MYTH: Chest pain is a "normal" part of aging.
FACT: Chest pain is not "normal"—no matter what your age. It is a warning that something is wrong. There are many underlying causes of chest pain in women, and heart disease is just one of them. Anxiety, depression, gallbladder problems, bronchitis, and common indigestion can also cause chest pain.

If you have chest pain, you owe it to yourself to have it properly evaluated by a physician. You may find that your chest pain is not life-threatening at all, and can be easily treated. If the pain is indeed caused by heart disease, you can take comfort in knowing that you caught the problem before having a life-threatening heart attack, and that there are plenty of things you can do to treat it. With proper treatment, you and your physician can prevent a heart attack from ever happening. Whatever you do, don't ignore this important warning sign from your body.

MYTH: Estrogen causes blood clots and heart attacks and should be avoided in order to prevent heart and circulatory problems.

FACT: Twenty years ago, oral contraceptives were believed to increase a woman's risk of heart disease significantly. Later studies implicated cigarette smoking as the major cause of this increased risk, not the estrogen and progestogen in the pills. Today's oral contraceptives contain much lower doses of estrogen and progestogen than older versions, and are considered safer than ever before. Questions remain, however, about the effects of oral contraceptives on such cardiovascular risk factors as cholesterol, blood coagulation, insulin and glucose metabolism, and blood pressure, particularly among older, premenopausal women, whose risk of heart disease naturally increases with age.

New studies—including studies at our clinic—have shown that the new low-dose oral contraceptives do not significantly raise a woman's risk of heart disease. In fact, birth control pills are now considered safe even for women over the age of forty. Nevertheless, if you are over forty, you should undergo a complete cardiovascular examination before taking oral contraceptives. You should also be monitored periodically while taking birth control pills to ensure that your risk isn't increased.

The results of the early studies on oral contraceptives were erroneously applied to postmenopausal hormonal preparations, which involve the use of much lower doses of estrogen that is chemically different from the estrogen used in birth control pills and that much more closely resembles the estrogen found in the human body. Only in the last ten years has new research demonstrated that postmenopausal estrogens actually protect against heart disease. *Numerous studies have demonstrated up to a 50 percent decreased risk of heart disease among postmenopausal women who take estrogen, as compared to nonusers.*

In addition, our own research and that of other scientists has found that postmenopausal estrogens may actually *lower* blood pressure. Research has found no evidence that postmenopausal estrogen preparations increase the likelihood of blood clots (one of the most common causes of heart attacks and strokes). Collectively, these findings are helping to make postmenopausal estrogens an important component of an overall program of prevention.

MYTH: A finger-prick cholesterol test is all you need to determine whether or not you are at risk of developing heart disease.

FACT: Although a finger-prick test can be an important first step in evaluating your risk of cardiovascular disease, the results should be interpreted carefully. As Deborah's story illustrated at the beginning of this chapter, it's possible to have "normal" total cholesterol levels and still be vulnerable to heart disease. In fact, up to 80 percent of people who have heart attacks have cholesterol levels within the normal range.

If you are past menopause, or if you have other risk factors for heart disease, regardless of your age, total cholesterol is not an adequate gauge of risk. Why not? To begin with, studies have found that high LDL cholesterol, low HDL cholesterol, and high triglycerides are all significant risk factors for heart disease in menopausal women. What this means is that you can have normal or mildly elevated total cholesterol, suggesting a fairly low risk; but, upon further testing, you may be found to have low HDL cholesterol, high triglycerides, or both. Therefore, you could be at a greater risk than the total cholesterol level suggests.

High LDL cholesterol can also be a problem. LDL cholesterol rises after menopause and should be carefully monitored. So finger-prick tests that reveal normal total cholesterol levels may give you a false sense of security.

In order to gauge your risk properly, you must have a blood test known as a *lipid profile*, which includes measures of total LDL and HDL cholesterol and triglycerides. Levels of these subfractions of cholesterol are much more accurate in determining risk than total cholesterol.

Another problem with *any* cholesterol test is that it doesn't take into account other factors that influence your risk of heart disease, such as family history, cigarette smoking, diet, and exercise patterns. All of these factors, together with cholesterol tests, must be evaluated in order to gauge your risk of heart disease. For this reason, it is best to work with your regular doctor to determine your individual risk profile.

MYTH: Women with heart disease receive the same medical treatment as men.

FACT: Don't count on it. Numerous studies have documented a serious "gender gap" in health care provided to women with heart disease. Generally speaking, heart disease is diagnosed at a later stage in women than in men, is more serious, and is treated less aggressively. For example, studies have found that women with coronary heart disease experience chest pain as their chief symptom more frequently than men. Yet fewer women than men are referred for appropriate diagnostic tests. Even when noninvasive tests suggest that significant coronary heart disease exists, fewer women than men are referred for the standard medical treatments: balloon angioplasty and coronary artery bypass surgery.

The gender gap in health care is partly a result of a gender gap in research that, in the past, has often excluded women from studies. For example, more than 10,000 men with preexisting heart disease have been enrolled in studies investigating the effectiveness of reducing blood cholesterol levels for the prevention of a second heart attack, compared with just over 400 women. Women of childbearing age are generally at such low risk that many researchers didn't think it was important for them to participate in studies. Elderly women typically were excluded from research because they are often plagued with other chronic illnesses that might adversely influence the study results.

As a result of all of this, many health care professionals succumbed to the same "heart-disease-can't-happen-to-women" myth as women themselves—and, in fact, may have helped to perpetuate that myth. In the past, when a woman went to her physician complaining of chest pain, she was likely to be evaluated for everything *but* heart disease, and was often (and often tragically) sent home with a pat on the back and an admonition that it was all in her head. But thanks to increased awareness of the problem by both women *and* their doctors, the situation is beginning to change.

MYTH: Advice and treatment regimens from studies based on men are equally good for women.
FACT: The scientific community is just beginning to recognize the fallacy of this kind of reasoning. For example, the Framingham, Massachusetts, Heart Study—one of the few studies to include women as research subjects—found that blood levels of *triglycerides* (fats circulating in the bloodstream) are an important barometer of increased risk of heart disease in women but not in men. Other studies have suggested that low HDL cholesterol (the "good" cholesterol that helps protect against heart disease) may be a more important risk factor for women than high LDL cholesterol (the "bad" cholesterol associated with an increased risk of heart attacks). What this means is that the guidelines for screening women for heart disease are somewhat different from those for men.

Researchers have also found that treatments that work well in men may not work equally well in women. More women than men die while undergoing coronary bypass surgery to restore blood flow to the heart muscle. Women also fare worse than men with less-invasive procedures for the treatment of artery-narrowing plaques, such as balloon angioplasty (use of a miniature balloon attached to a catheter to open clogged arteries) and atherectomy (surgical removal of a plaque from an artery). Studies have found that women don't get as much relief from their symptoms as do men undergoing the same procedures. Women also suffer more complications from the procedures than do men. No one knows yet whether women fare more poorly than men because of their smaller size, their more advanced age, the existence of other illnesses when they are diagnosed with cardiovascular disease, or because women receive less than adequate or delayed medical care. Whatever the reasons, these studies strongly suggest that the standard practice of basing advice to women on studies of men may be useless, and sometimes even dangerous.

Closing the Gender Gap

The good news is that the gender gap in research and in health care for cardiovascular disease is closing. More studies involving women are now underway. And more and more women are looking for information on how to protect themselves from cardiovascular disease.

Education is critical because *your risk of suffering a heart attack or stroke can be substantially reduced and a majority of premature deaths from cardiovascular disease prevented if medical intervention begins early.* Overall, preventive efforts in this country are already paying off: Over the past twenty years, the number of deaths due to cardiovascular disease has been cut in half, thanks to more advanced treatment and to increased public awareness of such risk factors as high blood pressure, cigarette smoking, and cholesterol. (Here again, however, women lag behind men. Since the 1950s, the rate of decline in deaths due to heart disease has fallen more slowly for women than for men.)

More good news: There is strong evidence that heart disease can be reversed in women as well as in men by lifestyle changes, certain medications, or a combination of both. In fact, the few preliminary studies involving women have found that *regression of artery-narrowing plaques occurs more readily in women, and the regression is more dramatic in women than in men.*

For Women Only

With the right information and the proper medical care, you *can* protect yourself from the leading cause of death of women today. The information you need to get the care you deserve is here, in *The Essential Heart Book for Women.* In this comprehensive book, you will find age-appropriate, gender-specific advice for women like you, based on the latest scientific research. In Part I, you'll see how a healthy heart works and how men and women differ in their heart profiles. In Part II, you'll find our complete program of prevention for coronary artery disease, the cause of most heart attacks in women. You'll learn about the special risk factors for women and the many ways in which you and your physician, working together, can reduce your risk through such healthier lifestyle habits as diet and exercise, and, if necessary, through drug therapy. You'll also find a thorough discussion of the critical role estrogen plays in the development and prevention of coronary artery disease. If you already have coronary artery disease, you'll learn what kind of treatment is available to you and what you can do to help prevent a heart attack. If you've already had a heart attack, you'll learn what to expect during your recovery and what you can do to prevent another one. Finally, in Part III, you'll find information on the causes, prevention, and treatment of other common forms of cardiovascular disease in women, including hypertension and stroke.

Studies have shown that an informed woman is better protected against cardiovascular disease. Why not begin your education here and now?

PART I

What Is Cardiovascular Disease?

CHAPTER 1

The Healthy Heart

YOUR CARDIOVASCULAR SYSTEM, consisting of your heart, lungs, and a vast network of blood vessels, is your body's life support system. Together, these organs are responsible for carrying oxygen and nutrients throughout your body and carrying away waste products. Without oxygen and nutrients, body tissues begin to die within minutes.

To understand what can go wrong—and what you can do to prevent future problems—it helps to have a basic understanding of how a healthy cardiovascular system works.

NOTE: If you are one of those people whose eyes gloss over at the thought of a lesson in basic anatomy, you can skip this section and still take the measures you need to protect yourself from heart disease. But if you are the type of woman who isn't satisfied following certain recommendations without knowing "why," you'll want to understand the information provided here.

The Heart: Nature's Perfect Pump

Your heart is one of the most important muscles in your body. The heart itself is only about the size of a clenched fist, but it is a workhorse. Every day, your heart, beating at an average rate of 60 to 70 beats per minute, pumps about 2,000 gallons of blood through some 58,000 miles of blood vessels.

Newly oxygenated blood from the lungs first fills the *left atrium*, the small chamber in the upper-left portion of the heart. Then, an electrical

FIGURE 1 — Anatomy of the Heart

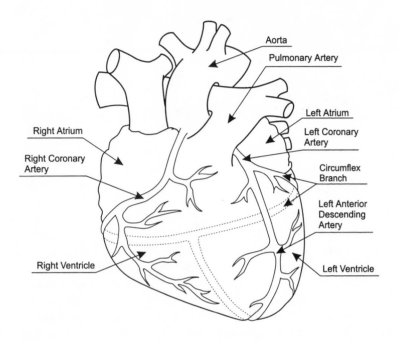

impulse causes the chamber to contract, opening up the *mitral valve* and pumping the blood into the larger lower-left chamber, known as the *left ventricle*. Again, an electrical impulse causes the chamber to contract, opening the aortic valve and ejecting the blood into large, thick-walled blood vessels called *arteries* (see Figure 1). Oxygen and nutrients in the blood flow through smaller and smaller arteries (*arterioles*) until they reach the *capillaries*, the tiniest blood vessels, measuring no more than a few cells wide. Here, the blood transfers oxygen and nutrients to virtually every cell in your body. The blood also carries away carbon dioxide and other waste products from the cells for disposal.

The blood travels back to the heart through a network of blood vessels called *veins*. It enters the *right atrium*, a small chamber in the upper-right portion of the heart, then is pumped into the *right ventricle* and finally back into the lungs, where it drops off carbon dioxide and picks up a fresh supply of oxygen. From there, the newly oxygenated blood is once again pumped through the left chambers of the heart and into the body.

Blood Vessels: Much More Than Basic Plumbing

The blood vessels themselves are much more than just "pipes" through which blood flows. They are organs in their own right, with their own internal control mechanisms to help move blood along, to prevent excessive bleeding, and to repair any damage should a blood vessel break or become injured. For example, the blood vessels can almost instantaneously dilate or contract as needed to regulate any sudden changes in blood flow or blood pressure, a characteristic known as *vascular tone*. The blood vessel walls also manufacture substances that aid in the formation of blood clots and that promote bleeding and prevent blood clots from forming. You'll learn more about the blood vessels and the critical role they play in the development of cardiovascular disease in Chapter 3.

Blood Pressure: The Great Equalizer

One of the main functions of the cardiovascular system is to maintain a steady supply of blood to all of the body's tissues at all times and under virtually any circumstances. This is accomplished by a finely tuned system of checks and balances that helps regulate blood pressure in the body.

Without the ability to regulate blood pressure almost instantaneously, the body would be unable to perform even the simple act of getting out of bed in the morning. When you sit or stand up, gravity pushes a large amount of blood toward your arms and legs. As a result, blood drains rapidly from the brain. If nothing is done to compensate for the shift in blood, you would pass out. Instead, the blood vessels in the arms and legs narrow to maintain adequate blood flow to the brain.

The body has a number of ways in which it regulates blood pressure. As mentioned earlier, the blood vessels have the capacity to dilate or constrict to adjust for rapid changes in blood flow and blood pressure. The heart itself can quickly adjust its output of blood as well, going from 60 to 70 beats per minute to up to 200 beats per minute as you sprint up a flight of stairs or make a mad dash for the commuter train.

While the heart and blood vessels can adapt to sudden changes in blood pressure, the body's fluid balance helps regulate blood pressure over longer periods of time—days, weeks, months, and years. This involves the kidneys, the amount of salt and water in the body, and hormones that help regulate the body's fluid balance.

The kidneys—the organs responsible for filtering waste materials from the blood—play a key role in regulating blood pressure over the long haul. When blood pressure rises, the kidneys respond by increasing their excretion of water and salt. This decreases the body's fluid volume *and* blood volume, thereby decreasing blood pressure. (This is the concept behind the use of diuretics, which are drugs that promote the excretion of urine in the treatment of high blood pressure.) When blood pressure falls too low, the kidneys decrease their output of water and salt, which promotes the accumulation of body fluids and raises blood pressure.

Blood pressure control also depends on a critical amount of salt and possibly other minerals (also known as electrolytes) in the body fluids. The amount of salt in the body is partly dependent on how much salt you consume in your diet. When you increase your salt intake, it stimulates the body's thirst center, making you drink extra amounts of water to dilute the salt to a normal concentration. This increases the body's fluid volume. It also stimulates the pituitary gland in the brain to excrete increased amounts of *antidiuretic hormone*, which causes the kidneys to hold on to the additional water rather than excrete it through urine. This helps explain why reducing your salt intake can sometimes help control blood pressure.

Blood Clots: Life Giving and Life Threatening

Your body's ability to form blood clots can save your life by preventing you from bleeding to death when a blood vessel is injured. But when a blood clot forms within a vital artery and blocks blood flow, it can trigger a life-threatening heart attack or stroke. This sophisticated system of blood flow (bleeding) and blood clotting is called *hemostasis*. Hemostasis is a complex process involving the blood vessel itself, specialized cells that circulate in the bloodstream, known as *platelets*, and dozens of *coagulation factors* and *anticoagulation factors* in the blood.

What Can Go Wrong?

As you can see, the cardiovascular system is one of the most sophisticated and complicated systems in the body. Not surprisingly, any of a number of problems can arise to undermine it. The heart muscle itself can enlarge and weaken, causing *congestive heart failure*. Problems can occur with the heart's electrical conduction system, causing *arrhythmias*, or irregular heart beats. The heart's valves can become diseased or damaged, resulting in conditions such as *mitral valve prolapse*. Sometimes an unborn baby's heart may not develop properly, causing *congenital heart defects*, such as

HOW A BLOOD CLOT FORMS

When a blood vessel is injured or broken, platelets begin sticking to the exposed collagen in the blood vessel wall. The collagen triggers a number of biochemical changes in the platelets that ultimately lead to the formation of a clot. The platelets begin producing *thromboxane A2,*a compound that increases their "stickiness" and constricts the blood vessel to help prevent excessive blood loss.

Other biochemical changes in the platelets trigger a chain reaction among several blood coagulation factors, ultimately resulting in the activation of *thrombin.* This powerful blood coagulant converts the coagulation factor *fibrinogen* into tough *fibrin* strands that hold the platelets together.

The blood vessel wall itself secretes compounds called *endothelins,* some of the body's most powerful blood vessel constrictors. Not much is known about the exact role of endothelins in the regulation of blood flow and the formation of blood clots. But we do know that blood levels of endothelins are elevated after a heart attack.

For every action, there is an equal and opposite reaction. *Anticoagulants* help ensure that your blood circulation isn't threatened by the formation of blood clots. The cells lining the blood vessel wall manufacture *prostacyclin*, a prostaglandin that keeps platelets from sticking together. Prostacyclin is also a powerful vasodilator, widening the blood vessel to maintain blood circulation. This anticoagulant works in direct opposition to thromboxane A2 and endothelins.

The blood vessel's ability to manufacture prostacyclin decreases with age and among people with diabetes or atherosclerosis. This means there may be a direct link between the production of prostacyclin in the blood vessel wall and its vulnerability to the development of blood clots or atherosclerosis.

More recently, scientists have discovered that the blood vessel wall also secretes *endothelium-derived relaxing factor* (EDRF), also known as nitric oxide, the body's own version of the widely used heart medication *nitroglycerin.* Nitroglycerin has been prescribed since the nineteenth century to widen the coronary arteries and relieve bouts of angina. Apparently, EDRF acts together a hole in the heart where there shouldn't be one. The blood vessels that nourish the heart can become diseased as well, a condition known as *coronary artery disease.*

The following pages describe some of the most common heart conditions among women.

Coronary Artery Disease

Although coronary artery disease (CAD) affects more men than women, it is the leading cause of death for women in America today. Coronary artery disease, often referred to as "coronary heart disease," has nothing to do with blockages of blood flow through the heart's four chambers, as some people might think. Rather, the condition occurs when the arteries that supply oxygen and nutrients to the heart muscle become narrowed or blocked (see Figure 2).

Some thickening and hardening of the arteries, a process called *arteriosclerosis*, is a part of normal aging. Far more insidious, however, is *atherosclerosis*, a type of arteriosclerosis in which deposits of fatty substances—cholesterol, cellular waste products, calcium, and fibrin (the tough fibers of a blood clot)—build up on the inner lining of the artery, forming a hard *plaque*. As plaques grow bigger, they reduce the flow of blood through the arteries.

FIGURE 2 — Narrowing of the Coronary Arteries Due to Plaque Buildup

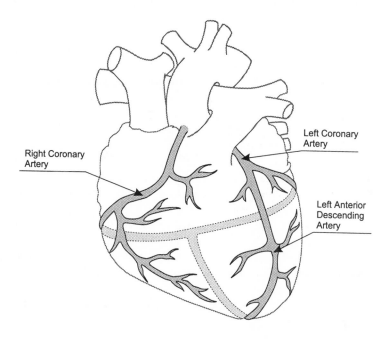

Left Coronary Artery

Right Coronary Artery

Left Anterior Descending Artery

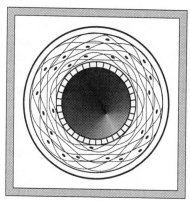

Normal Artery

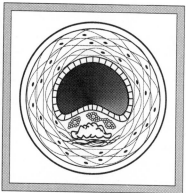

Artery with Atherosclerotic Plaque

The gradual narrowing of the coronary arteries reduces blood flow to the heart muscle, which can give rise to a number of heart conditions, including the following:

Angina

Angina is the medical term for chest pain resulting from restricted blood flow to the heart. The pain is a sign that the heart isn't getting enough oxygen. Angina is often triggered by strenuous activity (climbing stairs, for instance), extreme cold, or stress. The pain usually subsides when you rest, since a resting heart doesn't need as much oxygen as a working heart.

Chest pain is the most common symptom of heart disease in women. In the Framingham Heart Study, for instance, women were two times more likely to develop angina than to have a heart attack as their first symptom of heart disease. Unfortunately, chest pain is possibly the most misunderstood symptom by the medical community, mainly because so many other medical conditions can cause chest pain, for example, gastric reflux, gallbladder disease, panic attacks, and anxiety.

When blood flow to the heart is reduced, the resulting chest pain can be caused by something other than a buildup of plaque in the coronary arteries. For some reason, women are particularly susceptible to these other forms of angina. For instance, women are especially prone to a type of chest pain caused by spasms of coronary arteries that are apparently free of artery-narrowing plaques. This condition is known as *microvascular angina*.

Another type of chest pain in women with no evidence of atherosclerosis is thought to be caused by a decrease in the ability of the coronary arteries to dilate and contract as needed to regulate blood flow to the heart.

A disproportionate number of women also have *unstable angina*, which is chest pain that gets progressively worse over time and that doesn't respond well to treatment. A small percentage of men and women with unstable angina have normal coronary arteries; but, again, this condition is more likely to be found in women than in men.

Silent Ischemia

Silent ischemia is the term used to describe reduced blood flow to the heart that causes no pain. The danger is obvious: With no symptoms to warn of the condition, an affected woman may not get the medical attention she needs to treat it until it is too late. Unfortunately, no studies have examined gender differences in silent ischemia, so we don't know what percentage of women with heart disease have this condition.

IF YOU HAVE CHEST PAIN

Chest pain is one of the most frightening symptoms you can have, largely because it is a classic sign of a heart attack. But having chest pain doesn't necessarily mean you are having a heart attack or other serious heart problems. Chest pain can have any of a number of causes. Indigestion, anxiety, gallbladder disease, and menopausal hot flashes can cause chest discomfort, as can pneumonia, bronchitis, blood clots in the lungs, and such benign heart conditions as mitral valve prolapse. Moreover, many women experience chest pain and reduced blood flow to the heart with no signs of coronary artery disease, a condition known as *Syndrome X*. Of course, chest pain can be a sign of coronary artery disease, too. To make matters more confusing, many people who have a heart attack *don't* necessarily have chest pain.

In Chapter 12, you'll find an in-depth discussion of how to differentiate between the chest pain resulting from a heart attack and chest pain resulting from other causes. But take a few moments now to familiarize yourself with the warning signs of a heart attack.

You should immediately call for emergency help if you experience any of the following symptoms:

- An uncomfortable pressure, fullness, squeezing, or pain in the center of the chest that lasts longer than 15 minutes
- Severe chest pain
- Pain spreading to the shoulders, neck, or arms
- Lightheadedness and palpitations
- Fainting
- Sweating associated with chest discomfort
- Nausea associated with chest discomfort
- Difficulty breathing

Prompt medical attention may reduce the damage to your heart, and the more quickly you receive medical care, the greater your chances of surviving the attack.

Heart Attack

A heart attack, known in medical circles as a *myocardial infarction*, occurs when blood flow through a coronary artery becomes completely blocked, either through progressive narrowing (stenosis) of one or more coronary arteries, or when a blood clot (thrombosis) forms or gets lodged in a coronary artery. Sometimes a heart attack occurs when partially narrowed arteries go into spasm, temporarily reducing or cutting off blood flow to the heart tissue. With no oxygen and nutrients, the heart tissue supplied by the blocked artery begins to die, usually within thirty minutes of the time of blockage.

For many people, coronary artery disease exhibits no symptoms until a heart attack occurs. But this appears to be a bigger problem for men than for women. In the Framingham study, only 34 percent of women had a heart attack as their first symptom of coronary artery disease.

Unfortunately, when a woman does have a heart attack as her first symptom, it is more likely to be fatal. Thirty-nine percent of women versus 31 percent of men died of a first heart attack in the Framingham study. The long-term prognosis for women who survived the initial heart attack was also poorer than for men: 69 percent of these women died of coronary heart disease after one year, compared with 49 percent of men. For reasons that aren't yet clear, younger women (ages thirty-five to forty-four) and older women (ages seventy-five to eighty-four) in the Framingham study were most at risk of dying after a heart attack.

More women (35 percent) than men (27 percent) in the Framingham study also suffered a heart attack that went unrecognized. About half of these episodes in women were believed to have caused no symptoms, a condition known as a *silent myocardial infarction*. Symptomless heart attacks are more common in the elderly, particularly those with hypertension or diabetes.

Hypertension

If there's one type of heart disease that's an equal opportunity killer, it's hypertension, or high blood pressure. Half of the 50 million Americans with hypertension are women. And while researchers are not sure why, *after age forty-five, a woman's chances of having high blood pressure are greater than a man's.*

When you have high blood pressure, the arteries that help maintain blood pressure by dilating and contracting as needed remain constricted. As a result, your heart and arteries must strain to pump blood through your body. The heart may eventually enlarge and the arteries may become scarred, hardened, and less elastic.

The reduced blood flow means that other organs don't get the nutrients and oxygen they need. Your heart, brain, and kidneys are particularly susceptible to damage by high blood pressure. If left untreated, hypertension can lead to heart failure, stroke, and kidney damage. In fact, hypertension is the single most important modifiable risk factor for stroke as well as being a major risk factor for a heart attack.

Stroke

Stroke is another major cause of disability and death among women that can often be prevented. Overall, stroke is the third largest cause of death, after heart disease and cancer. While the incidence of stroke is higher in men than in women, more women than men died of a stroke in 1990, the latest year for which statistics are available. In addition to being a leading cause of death, stroke is the single largest cause of serious disability in the United States today.

A stroke occurs when the blood supply to the brain is disrupted, either by a blood clot or by excessive bleeding from a ruptured artery. When nerve cells in the affected area of the brain don't get the oxygen and nutrients they need, they begin to die within minutes. Hence, the part of the body controlled by these cells can't function either. The resulting tissue damage may cause severe losses of mental and bodily functions, and often even death.

Arrhythmias

Arrhythmias are irregularities in the heart's rate or rhythm. Arrhythmias can either cause the heart rate to speed up (*tachycardia*) or to slow down (*bradycardia*). Another type of abnormal heart rhythm is known as *premature beats*.

Some arrhythmias may be barely noticeable, causing a fluttering sensation in the neck or chest. Some may feel simply as though your heart "skipped a beat." Others may be so strong that they create a pounding sensation in the chest or a feeling that the heart is racing.

Generally speaking, most abnormal heart rhythms are more of an annoyance than a serious health problem. Some, however, are severe enough or last long enough to interfere with the heart's ability to pump blood efficiently. *Ventricular arrhythmias*, affecting the lower (ventricle) chambers of the heart, are the most serious. Ventricular arrhythmias can trigger ventricular fibrillations, in which the lower chambers of the heart quiver uncontrollably or stop beating altogether. This can lead to sudden cardiac death if not promptly treated with cardiopulmonary resuscitation (CPR). Fortunately, younger women are at a very low risk of ventricular arrhythmias. Women over age sixty-five, however, are at a greater risk. Women with existing heart disease, those who smoke cigarettes, have problems with alcohol, and/or have a history of psychiatric problems are also at risk.

Other Cardiovascular Conditions

Women are more likely than men to develop certain other heart conditions. These include the following:

Mitral Valve Prolapse

Mitral valve prolapse (MVP) occurs when one or both leaflets that make up the mitral valve billow up into the heart's atrial chamber, often resulting in a clicking sound, or heart murmur. Mitral valve prolapse sometimes causes blood to be regurgitated or spilled back into the atrial chamber.

For reasons unknown, mitral valve prolapse is more common in women than men, affecting about 5 to 6 percent of women, compared with 2 to 3 percent of men. Only rarely, however, does MVP lead to more serious heart problems.

Rheumatic Heart Disease

Rheumatic heart disease occurs when the heart valves become damaged by a disease process that begins with a strep throat. If not treated, the streptococcal infection develops into acute rheumatic fever, a condition that affects the connective tissues of the body, particularly the heart, joints, brain, or skin. When the heart tissue (usually the valves) becomes permanently damaged by rheumatic fever, it is called rheumatic heart disease. Although both men and women can develop rheumatic fever, it affects women about one and a half times as frequently as men.

As frightening as many of these conditions sound, you can take comfort in knowing that the most prevalent forms of cardiovascular disease among women—coronary artery disease, hypertension, and stroke—are also some of the most preventable and treatable.

Before discussing what you can do to protect yourself from these potential killers, let's take a closer look at some of the reasons most women are better protected against heart disease when they are younger, and what makes women more vulnerable to heart problems when they do occur.

CHAPTER 2

How Men and Women Are Different

IN TERMS OF its basic anatomy and function, the female heart is no different from the male heart. But there are some basic differences between men and women that have a major impact on how and when cardiovascular disease develops in women.

Physiological Differences

Throughout their lives, women have a distinct biological advantage over men. Even sperm containing the female X chromosome are heartier and tend to live longer than those containing the more fragile Y chromosome. Women today can expect to live an average of seven years longer than men. And the fact that women are relatively immune from heart disease for about ten years longer than men helps contribute to increased female longevity.

The Protective Power of Estrogen

This biological protection against heart disease is believed to be conferred, in large part, by the reproductive hormone estrogen, produced mainly by the ovaries. One of the many ways in which estrogen may protect women is that it keeps levels of harmful LDL cholesterol low. After menopause, when estrogen levels fall, LDL cholesterol rises an average of 25 points. In addition, estrogen receptors have been found in blood vessel walls and in the heart itself, suggesting that the hormone may have a direct influence on the heart and circulatory system. (For more on estrogen, see Chapter 9.)

Conversely, men's vulnerability to heart disease is believed to be caused in part by high levels of the male hormone testosterone circulating in the bloodstream. Testosterone is known to raise levels of "bad" LDL cholesterol and lower levels of protective HDL cholesterol.

What about other forms of estrogen, such as oral contraceptives and postmenopausal hormone therapy? Because these drugs are prescribed so freely (Premarin, a postmenopausal estrogen preparation, is one of the most widely prescribed drugs in America) and because past studies associated oral contraceptives with an increased risk of heart attack or stroke, many women are concerned about how these hormonal preparations affect their risk of cardiovascular disease. We now know that cigarette smoking, not hormones, was largely to blame for the increased risk of heart attacks and strokes found among women over age thirty-five who used oral contraceptives. More recent studies have vindicated oral contraceptives, and none has found any long-term increased risk of heart disease associated with their use. As for postmenopausal estrogens, mounting evidence has found that they confer protection against the most common and deadly form of cardiovascular disease in women: coronary artery disease.

Another important physiological difference between men and women is that throughout their lives, women have higher levels of protective HDL cholesterol, believed to help rid the body of excessive amounts of the "bad" LDL cholesterol. Even after menopause, when the drop in estrogen often triggers a rise in LDL cholesterol, levels of HDL cholesterol remain fairly constant. (See Table 2.)

What About Pregnancy?

Does pregnancy affect a woman's risk of developing heart disease? Pregnancy itself *does* put added stress on the cardiovascular system, but most healthy young women can handle the rigors of pregnancy with no adverse effects on their cardiovascular health. Some women with existing heart disease may have to take certain precautions during pregnancy, and those with severe heart conditions may be advised *not* to have children because a weakened heart cannot withstand the added stress of pregnancy.

Because blood lipids, insulin, and blood sugar levels rise sharply during pregnancy (they return to pre-pregnancy levels shortly after the baby is born), researchers have long wondered what effect, if any, pregnancy would have on a woman's long-term risk of developing heart disease. Past studies have been inconsistent, with some showing that pregnancy has a

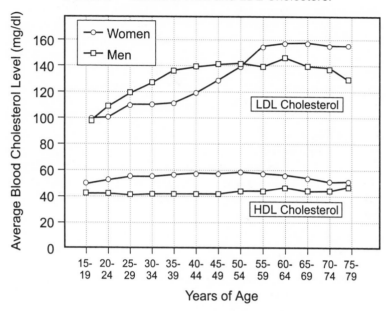

TABLE 2 — Levels of HDL and LDL Cholesterol

protective effect and others finding pregnancy to increase a woman's risk. Then in 1993, researchers gathered data from all 2,357 of the women who participated in the Framingham Heart Study for twenty-eight years, and from another 2,533 women ages forty-five to seventy-four enrolled in a government study (the National Health and Nutrition Examination Survey) for twelve years. They found that women who had been pregnant did have a slightly higher rate of coronary heart disease than those who had never been pregnant. But the risk was statistically significant *only* for women who had been pregnant six or more times. So unless you are planning (or already have) an extra-large family, pregnancy doesn't appear to increase your risk significantly.

Some Disadvantages of Being a Woman

One physiological difference that may not work in a women's favor is her smaller body size. A woman's heart and arteries are considerably smaller than a man's, so it takes less plaque to slow or completely disrupt blood flow through a woman's blood vessels.

The loss of estrogen after menopause takes a toll, too. Women whose menopause occurs early (before age thirty-five) have a two- to threefold increased risk of heart attack, and those whose estrogen-producing ovaries are surgically removed before age thirty-five have a sevenfold increased risk. As we mentioned earlier, LDL cholesterol rises an average of 25 points after menopause, which contributes to the increased risk of heart disease among postmenopausal women. But the lack of estrogen may adversely affect a woman's risk of heart disease in other ways as well (see Chapter 9).

Because women tend to be older than men when they are first diagnosed with heart disease, their advanced age also works against them. This is partly because older bodies are more fragile and slower to heal. In addition, while women tend to live longer than men, they are often plagued with chronic health conditions later in life, such as diabetes or hypertension. Too often, cardiovascular disease is just one of a number of health problems with which older women have to contend.

Other Differences

Together, these physiological differences—smaller body size, loss of protection by estrogen at the time of menopause, more advanced age at the time of diagnosis, and the coexistence of other health problems—may all contribute to a poorer prognosis for women with cardiovascular disease. But most scientists agree that the physiological differences between the sexes don't entirely explain why women with heart disease don't fare as well as men.

Changing Social Roles

Women's social roles have changed tremendously over the past forty years. More and more women today are working, and there's a general concern that they are now exposed to the same physical and emotional hazards of the work environment as men. Would the increased stress result in an increased risk of heart disease?

Research has found that in men, the competitive, hard-driving Type A personality often associated with success is also associated with an increased risk of heart disease. While the research on Type A behavior in women is still in its infancy, many experts worry that women with these personality traits may also be at a greater risk of developing heart disease.

Perhaps more important is the fact that many women today—especially those with young children—now juggle work and family roles simultaneously, creating role conflicts and overload. And women appear to handle this role overload differently from men. For instance, research from the University of Stockholm has found that rather than "unwinding" after returning home from work in the evening as men do, women continue to exhibit increased cardiovascular arousal, suggesting that women continue their "workday" in the home environment.

Other experts point to increased substance abuse among women over the past several decades, suggesting another way that women cope with the added stress of role overload. Substance abuse can substantially increase a woman's risk of heart disease.

Some researchers speculate that these social changes may help explain why death rates for cardiovascular disease have not fallen as rapidly for women as they have for men over the past twenty years.

Lack of Social Support
Another possible explanation for the poorer prognosis among women diagnosed with heart disease is social isolation. Because women tend to be older when they are diagnosed with heart disease, they often have outlived their spouses and are likely to be living alone. Studies have found that the risk of having a second heart attack is greater for women living alone than for those with more social supports.

Economic Differences
Some groups of women, especially elderly and minorities, may not have as good access to health care because of economic woes. Poor elderly make 25 percent fewer visits to the doctor compared with people whose income is 200 percent above poverty level. Moreover, black and poor elderly are less likely to have private health insurance to supplement Medicare coverage, and are less likely to receive preventive care services.

Differences in Health Care
A lack of money or health insurance isn't the only barrier to good medical care for women with heart disease. Remember that research has found that a gender bias by the medical community exists as well, possibly fueled by the myth that heart disease is a "man's" problem. In one study, researchers investigated the way doctors responded to five medical complaints common in both men and women: chest pain, back pain, headache, dizziness, and fatigue. Men received a more extensive workup than women for all complaints, suggesting that men with symptoms are taken more seriously than women with symptoms. Another study found that ten men

were referred for cardiac catheterization after an abnormal screening test to every one woman.

Women also tend to be less aggressively treated for heart disease than men. In the Coronary Artery Surgery Study (CASS), for example, women were referred for coronary artery bypass surgery much later in the course of their disease than men. The National Heart, Lung and Blood Institute also found similar differences between men and women referred for coronary angioplasty (widening of the coronary arteries by a balloon attached to a catheter).

It is still not clear why these gender biases in treatment exist. Some say that fewer women are referred for cardiac procedures because of concern about higher mortality rates in women undergoing bypass surgery. It's also possible that the higher death rates among women with heart disease are the result of delays in the proper diagnosis and treatment.

Whatever the reason for the gender bias in the diagnosis and treatment of heart disease, you can help put a stop to it. Your best defense is knowledge. Read on to find out how you can prevent coronary artery disease, the leading cause of death of American women today.

PART II

Coronary Artery Disease

CHAPTER 3

How Coronary Artery Disease Develops

IN SIMPLEST TERMS, coronary artery disease is a buildup of hard plaques on the walls of the coronary arteries, which supply oxygen and nutrients to the heart muscle. But the way this happens is anything but simple.

You've undoubtedly heard that cholesterol, the fatty substance that circulates in your bloodstream, is a major contributor to coronary heart disease. And with all the talk about cholesterol in recent years, you may have been led to believe it was the *only* cause. But cholesterol is just one of many contributing factors to the development of coronary artery disease, and watching your dietary cholesterol intake is just one of many approaches you can take to prevent it. More recently, researchers have begun focusing on the role of your body's ability to make (and dissolve) blood clots, the role of insulin, and the role of the immune system (see Figure 3). And, of course, there's estrogen, which is now known to *protect* women from coronary heart disease in the premenopausal years. As you'll see in later chapters, a family history of premature heart disease and such lifestyle factors as cigarette smoking, lack of exercise, poorly controlled diabetes, unchecked hypertension, and stress also play a part. With a basic understanding of how and why the disease develops, you'll have a better grasp of the whys and wherefores of prevention and treatment— and you might just be more motivated to take action.

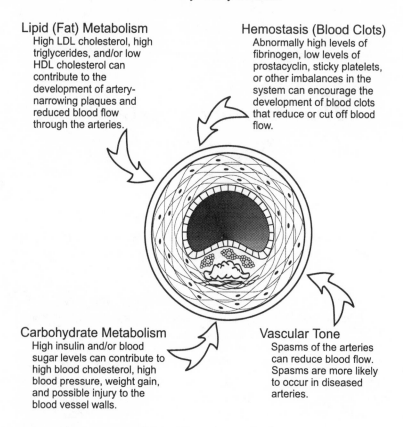

FIGURE 3 — Four Underlying Causes of Coronary Artery Disease

Lipid (Fat) Metabolism
High LDL cholesterol, high triglycerides, and/or low HDL cholesterol can contribute to the development of artery-narrowing plaques and reduced blood flow through the arteries.

Hemostasis (Blood Clots)
Abnormally high levels of fibrinogen, low levels of prostacyclin, sticky platelets, or other imbalances in the system can encourage the development of blood clots that reduce or cut off blood flow.

Carbohydrate Metabolism
High insulin and/or blood sugar levels can contribute to high blood cholesterol, high blood pressure, weight gain, and possible injury to the blood vessel walls.

Vascular Tone
Spasms of the arteries can reduce blood flow. Spasms are more likely to occur in diseased arteries.

The Role of Cholesterol

We've known for some time that the development of plaques is strongly associated with high levels of *cholesterol* circulating in your blood. Cholesterol is a fatty substance found in meat and dairy products and in every cell in your body, where it is used to form cell membranes that help carry out the cell's basic functions. Cholesterol also helps manufacture certain hormones, notably estrogen and vitamin D. Indeed, cholesterol is so essential to your survival that *your liver manufactures virtually all the cholesterol you need.*

But there's much more to the cholesterol story than the "good" high-density lipoproteins and "bad" low-density lipoproteins you may be familiar with. When we talk about cholesterol, we're actually referring to several different types of fat and cholesterol, collectively known as *blood lipids*. Since fat and water don't mix, the liver pairs up fat and cholesterol with protein carriers called *apolipoproteins* so they can be transported in the bloodstream and deposited into cells. The resulting particles are known as *lipoproteins*. Each has a role in your body's processing and handling of fat and cholesterol—and many are involved in the development of atherosclerosis.

Triglycerides

In simplest terms, triglycerides are a form of fat your body can use. The liver makes some of the triglycerides circulating in your bloodstream. Fats in the foods you eat are also broken down in the small intestine and converted to triglycerides, to be used for energy or stored as fat.

It's still not clear what role triglycerides play in the development of heart disease. Certain forms of abnormally high triglyceride levels, which are caused by a genetic flaw (a condition known as *familial hypertriglyceridemia*), are associated with narrowing of the arteries at a much earlier age than expected. Thus we know that high triglycerides can promote the development of atherosclerosis. Other researchers have found an association between high triglycerides and increased activity of certain blood coagulants, suggesting that triglycerides may encourage the development of blood clots as well.

The research on high triglycerides and coronary risk has been inconsistent in men, which may help explain why the medical community hasn't placed much emphasis on treating high triglycerides. Researchers associated with the Framingham Heart Study, however, report that elevated triglycerides are a powerful predictor of coronary heart disease in women over age fifty. This is particularly true when high triglycerides (above 300 mg/dl) are combined with low levels of HDL cholesterol (below 40 mg/dl).

Triglyceride levels are determined partly by the amount of fat in the foods you eat (most of the fat in our diets is triglyceride), partly by the amount of refined carbohydrates you eat ("sugar fats"), and partly by your genes. Triglycerides also rise with age. Being overweight can raise triglyceride levels, as can non-insulin-dependent diabetes, oral contraceptives, and oral postmenopausal estrogens.

Very-Low-Density Lipoproteins

These fat particles, manufactured by the liver, are laden with triglycerides. They also contain some cholesterol. Their chief role is to carry triglycerides to the muscles for energy and to fat tissues for storage.

Again, we don't know the precise role of VLDL in development of heart disease. Animal studies, however, have shown that an unusual form of small, dense VLDL, known as *beta-VLDL*, is involved in the development of artery-clogging plaques.

Low-Density Lipoproteins

After their cargo has been delivered, the VLDL break up into smaller particles containing mostly cholesterol. These are known as *low-density lipoproteins* (LDL), whose chief role is to transport cholesterol to your cells. Some of the LDL is also returned to the liver, where it can be broken down and cleared from the body.

LDL cholesterol truly does live up to its reputation as the "bad" cholesterol; this is the type of cholesterol that accumulates on the artery walls, helping to form artery-narrowing plaques.

New research has demonstrated that LDL cholesterol must somehow become "damaged" before it can develop into a plaque. Many researchers now are convinced that *oxidation* of the LDL molecules by *oxygen free radicals* is one of the main culprits. Free radicals are highly charged particles that are missing one electron. They are naturally occurring by-products of metabolism in your body, and are also formed by certain drugs, cigarette smoking, excessive sun exposure, and some substances in foods. Essentially, free radicals bombard the fat particle, thus adding an extra oxygen molecule to the chain of molecules that make up LDL cholesterol. When this happens, the oxidized LDL cholesterol is more likely to be deposited on artery walls.

In addition, there are several subtypes of LDL cholesterol believed to be more or less atherogenic. For instance, studies have shown that high levels of a small, densely packed cholesterol molecule, known as *small-molecule LDL* cholesterol, are associated with a threefold increased risk of heart attack.

LDL cholesterol levels rise after menopause, which may help explain why postmenopausal women are more vulnerable to heart disease.

High-Density Lipoproteins

High-density lipoproteins (HDL), which are manufactured in the small intestine and the liver, are believed to haul cholesterol back to the liver for processing and disposal. HDL cholesterol may even help remove cholesterol deposits from the artery walls, which is why it is often referred to as the "good" cholesterol. There are two main types of HDL cholesterol:

HDL$_2$ and HDL$_3$. HDL$_3$ is believed to be a precursor of HDL$_2$. High levels of HDL cholesterol help protect against heart disease.

As with the other lipids circulating in your bloodstream, levels of HDL cholesterol are determined partly by your genes and partly by such lifestyle factors as your weight, how much you exercise, the amount of alcohol you consume, and whether you smoke cigarettes. Women generally have higher levels of HDL cholesterol than men, which may help explain the lower incidence of heart disease among women, at least until after menopause, when levels of LDL cholesterol rise.

Ironically, it appears that you may need *some* fat in your diet for your body to manufacture HDL cholesterol. A study by British researchers found that while exercise raised levels of HDL cholesterol, the effects of exercise on HDL cholesterol levels were greater when study participants ate a diet moderately high in fat.

Apolipoproteins

These are the protein carriers of fat and cholesterol in the bloodstream. Several different types of apolipoproteins have been identified, and all are receiving increased scrutiny in their role in the development of, and protection from coronary heart disease. Apolipoprotein A is the protein carrier of HDL cholesterol. Apo B carries LDL cholesterol through the bloodstream.

Of particular interest in recent years is a newly discovered particle called apolipoprotein (a) (pronounced "apolipoprotein little-a"). Researchers have found that high blood levels of apolipoprotein (a) are associated with an increased risk of heart attacks among people with a genetic predisposition to dangerously high blood cholesterol levels, a condition known as *familial hypercholesterolemia.*

Elevated cholesterol and triglyceride levels are just some of many factors that contribute to coronary artery disease. In fact, many people with elevated cholesterol levels don't have a heart attack. And up to 80 percent of people who have heart attacks *don't* have high cholesterol. The reason, as we mentioned earlier, is that high cholesterol is only one of many contributing factors to heart disease.

The Role of Blood Clots

The formation of blood clots in the arteries plays such a critical role in coronary artery disease that the condition might be more appropriately named *atherothrombosis* (a thrombosis is a blood clot that lodges in a major artery). As you may recall from Chapter 1, hemostasis is a complex process involving blood cells known as *platelets*, and numerous coagulants and anticoagulants.

Normally, platelets circulate freely in the blood vessels, and don't stick to the blood vessel wall unless it becomes injured. Problems begin when the body perceives the accumulation of fat on the artery wall as an injury. In an attempt to heal the wound, it often forms blood clots.

Small blood clots may actually become a part of the hard artery-narrowing plaque. Larger ones may contribute to the plaque's obstruction of blood flow. In fact, blood clots are one of the main causes of heart attacks.

Scientists have recently discovered what appears to be a critical link between cholesterol metabolism and the body's blood clotting system: As it turns out, apolipoprotein (a) is closely related in chemical structure to the anticoagulant plasminogen produced by the blood vessel wall. They suspect that apolipoprotein (a) somehow competes with plasminogen after a clot begins forming in a blood vessel wall. If apolipoprotein (a) gets the upper hand, it short-circuits the blood vessel's natural ability to dissolve the clot.

As you can see, blood coagulation plays a key role in the development of heart attacks and strokes. Fortunately, as you'll learn in the chapters to come, there are ways to influence your body's system of hemostasis and further reduce your risk of cardiovascular disease. Over the last ten years, powerful clot-busting drugs, such as *streptokinase*, *urokinase*, and tPA (*tissue plasminogen activator*), have become crucial in the treatment of heart attacks, and can even stop a heart attack in progress. You can also see how aspirin, which affects platelets, can be used to help prevent heart attacks and strokes.

The Role of Insulin

It is probably no coincidence that people with diabetes also have high blood cholesterol levels, often develop hypertension, and are at an increased risk of cardiovascular disease. We're just beginning to recognize the importance of insulin in the development of hypertension and athero-sclerosis, a condition referred to as *Syndrome X* (not to be confused with another condition known as microvascular angina that is also referred to as Syndrome X and that is characterized by unexplained chest pain).

Insulin is a hormone produced by the pancreas that helps regulate blood sugar levels. After eating a meal or snack, the pancreas releases insulin into the bloodstream, where it helps sugar and fat from the food you eat enter your body's cells.

How can elevated insulin levels contribute to high blood pressure? The link appears to be the *sympathetic nervous system*, which regulates your heart rate, blood pressure, blood flow, metabolism, and other involuntary body functions. Insulin stimulates the adrenal glands to release the hormones *epinephrine* and *norepinephrine* into the bloodstream. These two hormones can raise your heart rate and blood pressure. High insulin levels also cause the kidneys to retain salt, which also raises blood pressure.

Insulin has been implicated in aiding and abetting the development of atherosclerosis, too. High blood sugar levels are believed to damage or alter the lining of the artery wall, allowing insulin to interact with the underlying tissues, and making them more sensitive to the development of fatty streaks and, ultimately, artery-narrowing plaques. To add insult to injury, insulin is also associated with high triglycerides and lower levels of protective HDL cholesterol.

Women with diabetes are most likely to have high blood sugar levels, high insulin levels, or both, which causes these women to lose their natural biological protection against heart disease.

The Role of the Immune System

Scientists are just beginning to understand the role of the body's immune defense system in the development of atherosclerosis. Most of the time, your immune defense system helps to keep foreign invaders, such as bacteria and viruses, at bay. But sometimes the immune system can contribute to the development of illnesses.

Monocytes and Macrophages
Key players in the formation of artery-clogging plaques are *monocytes*, a type of disease-fighting white blood cell. Monocytes transform into *macrophages*, scavenger cells that reside in certain tissues of the body and circulate in the bloodstream, where they gobble up bacteria and other foreign invaders much like the roving character in the video arcade game Pac Man.

When they take up residence in the artery wall just below the surface of the innermost layer (endothelium), macrophages attract and consume LDL cholesterol. Macrophages are particularly fond of oxidized (damaged)

LDL cholesterol, taking it up at a much faster rate than "native" (undamaged) LDL cholesterol.

The more LDL cholesterol the macrophages ingest, the more heavily loaded they become with fat droplets. When this happens, the macrophages transform into *foam cells* in the artery wall. If enough foam cells accumulate in one spot, they form a *fatty streak*. Fatty streaks, as you may recall, are the precursors of plaques.

Macrophages do their dirty work in other ways as well. The immune cells also produce toxic substances that may damage the cells lining the blood vessel wall. These toxic substances are thought to contribute to the oxidation (damage) of LDL cholesterol, too. In addition, macrophages secrete substances that stimulate the growth of smooth-muscle cells, which encapsulate the plaque. Macrophages can also release chemicals that promote the development of blood clots in and on the plaque.

Mast Cells

Another type of immune defense cell that may have a role in the development of atherosclerosis is the mast cell. Mast cells have long been considered "nuisance cells" of the body's immune defense system because of their involvement in allergy attacks—an overwhelming response of the immune system to a harmless substance, such as pollen.

Mast cells are manufactured in bone marrow and reside in various tissues throughout the body, chiefly the skin, respiratory passages (the nose, breathing tube, and lungs), the gastrointestinal tract, and adjacent to blood vessels, and throughout the body's lymphatic system. When activated by some kind of irritating substance, mast cells release a chemical known as *histamine*, which causes tissue cells to swell and become inflamed. Histamine is responsible for the skin inflammation that occurs around a bee sting, and for the sneezing, runny nose, and watery eyes that occur when an allergy sufferer is exposed to an airborne allergen, such as ragweed pollen. Histamine and *serotonin*, another substance released by the mast cell, also constrict blood vessels and increase the heart rate.

Vanderbilt University researchers have already found that as arterial lesions progress toward becoming plaques, the number of mast cells in the outer layers of the arterial wall increases, as does the amount of histamine in the lesions. Although more research needs to be conducted, they think that mast cells may promote inflammation of the cells in the blood vessel walls, which, in turn, attracts monocytes to the area and promotes the development of fatty streaks.

Heat Shock Proteins

Another hint that the body's immune defense system plays a role in the development of atherosclerosis comes from a recent study published in the prestigious British medical journal the *Lancet*. Researchers found that people with plaque deposits in their arteries had a higher level of antibodies to *heat shock proteins*. These proteins are manufactured in large amounts by cells exposed to such assaults as heat or oxygen free radicals, or in response to certain substances produced by the immune system.

Antibodies to heat shock proteins have been detected in several inflammatory and autoimmune diseases (in which the body's immune defense system attacks its own tissues), such as rheumatoid arthritis, systemic lupus erythematosus, and insulin-dependent diabetes. Heat shock proteins have been associated with atherosclerosis as well. In fact, the British researchers found that the presence of antibodies to heat shock proteins was a strong, independent risk factor for atherosclerosis, statistically of the same magnitude as blood cholesterol and blood pressure.

The researchers suspect that the tissue damage caused by artery-narrowing plaques may trigger the production of heat shock proteins. These proteins, in turn, may provoke the immune defense system to make antibodies to them, resulting in an autoimmune response, in which the body's immune system mistakenly attacks its own tissues. They think the heat shock proteins may not be a cause of atherosclerosis, but the body's natural response to it.

The researchers note that there are similarities between heat shock proteins produced by the human body and by bacteria. It is possible that the body's production of antibodies to its own heat shock proteins could initially be directed against bacteria. If so, it's possible that microorganisms may be the cause of atherosclerosis.

In the meantime, a blood test that detects antibodies to heat shock proteins may become instrumental in helping to diagnose people with atherosclerosis. The presence of antibodies to heat shock proteins would signal a greater likelihood of diseased arteries, and the need for further diagnostic tests.

The Role of the Artery Wall

Before plaques can take hold, researchers now believe, the inner walls of the artery must somehow become injured. Even something as simple as a disturbance in the pattern of blood flow can cause minor injury to the endothelium, the delicate layer of cells that line the inner walls of the artery. In animals, high cholesterol levels, chemicals that dilate or contract the blood vessels, certain substances produced by the immune system, infection, and chemical irritants in tobacco smoke can injure the endothelium. The excessive force of blood pressure on the artery walls associated with hypertension can also damage the delicate inner lining of the artery, as can high levels of glucose (blood sugar) and insulin in people with diabetes.

Putting It All Together: The Development of the Plaque

Once the endothelium is injured, the stage is set for the development of a plaque (see Figure 4): The cells become inflamed, attracting monocytes to the injury. Monocytes are then transformed into macrophages, which attract lipids and form foam cells. Macrophages also release toxic substances, which damage the deeper tissues of the blood vessel wall. When this happens, platelets begin to adhere to the injury site in an attempt to heal the wound. Macrophages and platelets, together with the blood vessel wall itself, may release substances that fuel the growth of smooth-muscle cells, which encapsulate the plaque. These cells can be easily disrupted, leading to the formation of blood clots on the outside of the plaque. When blood clots are small, they can cause further damage to the middle layer of the blood vessel wall (the media) and fuel the growth of the plaque. When blood clots are large, they can partially or totally block the artery, causing such symptoms as angina or a heart attack.

When plaques build up on the inside of the artery wall, they interfere with the artery's ability to dilate and contract as needed to help regulate blood flow. As a result, diseased arteries are more likely than healthy arteries to develop spasms. Spasms are particularly dangerous in diseased arteries because they can cause a serious (though temporary) reduction in blood flow through the arteries (see Figure 5 on page 44).

The Role of Estrogen

Estrogen is believed to help protect women from developing heart disease in their reproductive years. The hormone is also credited with protecting postmenopausal women from developing heart and blood vessel diseases. How does estrogen protect?

Much of what we know about estrogen's ability to protect against

FIGURE 4 — How Plaque Forms

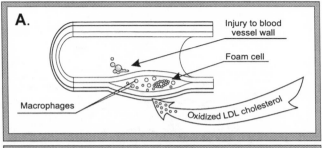

A. Injury to blood vessel wall
Foam cell
Macrophages
Oxidized LDL cholesterol

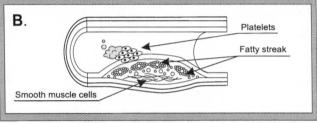

B. Platelets
Fatty streak
Smooth muscle cells

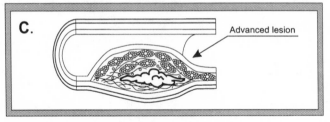

C. Advanced lesion

A. Injury to blood vessel wall, possibly due to:
   • high blood pressure
   • high insulin levels
   • high blood cholesterol levels
   • inflammation
   • illness
   Macrophages (white blood cells) accumulate at the site of injury, attracting LDL cholesterol. Oxidized LDL cholesterol molecules infiltrate the blood vessel wall and, together with macrophages, form foam cells.

B. Clusters of foam cells form fatty streaks in the artery walls. Platelets adhere to the injury, releasing growth factors that cause excessive growth of cells in smooth muscle of the artery.

C. The result is an advanced lesion that reduces blood flow through the artery.

FIGURE 5 — How Artery Spasms Reduce Blood Flow

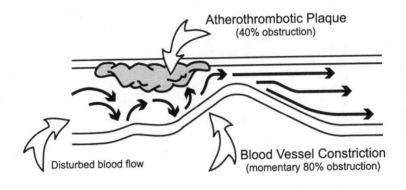

Atherothrombotic Plaque
(40% obstruction)

Disturbed blood flow

Blood Vessel Constriction
(momentary 80% obstruction)

heart disease comes from studies on oral contraceptives, postmenopausal estrogen preparations, and the effects of menopause and surgical menopause on a woman's risk of heart disease. For instance, we know that estrogens have a powerful effect on blood lipids and lipoproteins. Total cholesterol levels rise an average of 25 points after menopause when the ovaries' production of estrogen declines. This translates into roughly a 50 percent increase in a woman's risk of developing heart disease.

Moreover, women who take postmenopausal oral estrogens experience a decline in total and LDL cholesterol and a rise in protective HDL$_2$ cholesterol. The change in blood lipids depends on the amount of estrogen you take: the higher the dose, the greater the change. On average, women who take the higher dose of 1.25 milligrams of conjugated equine oral estrogens per day experience a rise in HDL cholesterol of 14 to 17 percent, while LDL cholesterol falls an average of 8 percent. In a study we conducted on the effects of oral estrogens on blood lipids, women taking 1.25 milligrams of estrogen (estropipate) daily experienced nearly a 10 percent increase in HDL cholesterol after twelve months, an 8 percent drop in LDL cholesterol, and a marked improvement in the ratios of HDL to LDL cholesterol and total cholesterol to HDL cholesterol.

Estrogens appear to protect your heart in other ways as well. Contrary to popular belief, estrogens *don't* raise blood pressure, as early studies involving oral contraceptives once suggested. In the Postmenopausal Estrogen-Progestin Interventions (PEPI) Trial, the largest and most carefully controlled study to date on the effects of postmenopausal hormonal preparations on heart disease risk factors, blood pressure was unaffected by postmenopausal hormones. And several small studies have found that oral postmenopausal estrogen preparations can actually *decrease* blood pressure. In a study at our clinic, estrogens alone decreased blood pressure by an average of 3.8 percent.

What about blood clots? It's still not clear what effect estrogen has on the formation of blood clots. It's true that the risk of *thromboembolism* (the formation of one or more blood clots in the deep veins of the legs) increases during pregnancy, when estrogen and progesterone levels are high. Oral contraceptives—particularly the older pills, which contained much higher doses of estrogen than today's—have been associated with an increased risk of blood clots. But as the doses of estrogen in oral contraceptives have decreased, so has the incidence of blood clots that develop in the veins (venous blood clots). In a recent study, we investigated the effects of low-dose oral contraceptives on certain coagulants and anticoagulants in the blood that govern the development of these blood clots. We found that the changes the hormone had on blood coagulants were balanced by changes in anticoagulants. So the new low-dose oral contraceptives appear to have a minimal effect on the development of venous thrombosis—(blood clots in the veins).

While the risk of developing arterial blood clots (the kind that can precipitate a heart attack or stroke) is very low among oral contraceptive users, these types of blood clots do occasionally occur. We don't fully understand how or why these blood clots develop. In the past, estrogen was suspected of increasing the stickiness of platelets, thus increasing the risk of developing a blood clot. Recent studies have demonstrated that just the opposite occurs: Estrogen actually *decreases* the stickiness of platelets.

What about postmenopausal estrogen preparations, which are chemically different from the synthetic estrogens in birth control pills, and are given in much lower doses than oral contraceptives? While oral postmenopausal estrogens *do* increase the liver's production of several different coagulants, these substances are not biologically active until they're exposed to an injured blood vessel. Plus, "normal" levels for many of these coagulation factors vary widely, and it's impossible to predict who is at higher risk of developing blood clots by measuring levels of these enzymes. What's more, the PEPI Trial found that women who took hormones had lower levels of the blood coagulant fibrinogen than women who took a placebo. Fibrinogen is an independent risk factor for both heart attacks and strokes, and the lower fibrinogen levels among hormone users suggests that postmenopausal hormones may protect in a variety of ways.

On the other hand, we found that postmenopausal estrogens *don't have any effect at all* on anticoagulants, particularly antithrombin III, which is a good marker for predicting whether you will develop a blood clot. In addition, we've found that menopause itself raises levels of potential anticlotting factors, such as plasminogen, possibly providing some natural protection against the formation of blood clots. This may help explain why postmenopausal estrogen therapy appears less likely to cause blood clots in older women. Indeed, *there is no study showing a cause-and-effect relationship between taking estrogen therapy and the development of blood clots.* Estrogen's poor reputation comes from studies on the use of older, high-dose oral contraceptives among older women who smoked. *Smoking is the demon!*

As for insulin, estrogen *decreases* fasting blood sugar levels, possibly because it prevents the breakdown of insulin. This may provide added protection against heart disease.

Estrogens may protect in other ways as well. For instance, estrogen stimulates the artery walls to release a substance known as EDFR (nitric oxide), which dilates the arteries. Estrogen also inhibits the release of *endothelin*, a substance that constricts the arteries. And estrogen also directly affects the smooth muscle tissue underneath the lining of the artery, helping to relax the artery. The end result is increased blood flow, which increases the delivery of oxygen and nutrients to the body's tissues.

The hormone also appears somehow to protect the innermost lining of the blood vessel wall, where artery-narrowing plaques form. At least three studies have shown that postmenopausal women who take estrogens are less likely to have occluded arteries than women who don't use estrogen. Angiograms, in which a dye is injected into the bloodstream and an X ray is taken as the dye passes through the coronary arteries, showed that estrogen users had significantly less stenosis (narrowing) than nonusers, even when other risk factors, including hypertension, diabetes, cigarette smoking, and obesity, were taken into account. Indeed, estrogens appeared to reduce the risk of severe coronary artery disease by a striking 56 to 63 percent. Estrogen has antioxidant properties, which may help prevent the damage to the artery wall that makes it vulnerable to the development of plaques. Estrogen also helps keep LDL cholesterol from oxidation. (Oxidized LDL cholesterol plays a major role in the development of atherosclerosis.)

Animal studies also suggest that estrogens somehow protect against atherosclerosis. In a study conducted by Dr. Thomas B. Clarkson and colleagues at Wake Forest University in North Carolina, monkeys who were fed a high-fat diet and given oral contraceptives were expected to have a twofold increase in the extent of coronary narrowing. Instead, the monkeys were found to have 50 to 75 percent *less* atherosclerosis—*in spite of the fact that the birth control pills lowered levels of protective HDL cholesterol.* The researchers believe that the estrogen in oral contraceptives somehow protects the coronary arteries from the development of artery-narrowing plaques.

A Lifelong Process

Atherosclerosis doesn't just happen overnight. Rather, it is a gradual process that takes years—possibly half a lifetime or more—to develop. Researchers studying heart disease risks among children in the town of Bogalusa, Louisiana, found that *children as young as age ten have fatty streaks in their arteries that are believed to develop later into artery-clogging plaques.* A major new study that includes men as well as women has confirmed the Bogalusa findings. The new study, known as the Pathobiological Determinants of Atherosclerosis in Youth (PDAY) study, found that atherosclerosis begins in childhood, and that the process increases rapidly in men and women between the ages of fifteen and thirty-four.

Obviously, the earlier medical intervention begins, the more likely you will be to prevent atherosclerosis from taking hold. And because the development of atherosclerosis is a complex process, one that involves much more than high cholesterol levels, your program of prevention should include a variety of measures. In the chapters that follow, we'll look at the various risk factors for atherosclerosis, and how you can lower your risk through modification of such lifestyle habits as your diet and exercise patterns.

CHAPTER 4

Are You at Risk?

SOME WOMEN are more vulnerable to developing coronary artery disease than others. If you have one or more of the risk factors discussed in this chapter, you may be one of those women. The good news is that many risk factors are within your control, and, by influencing them, you can substantially reduce your risk.

Major Risk Factors

The association between the following risk factors and an increased incidence of heart disease has been well established.

Your Age

Your risk of developing heart disease increases as you grow older. This is especially true of women. In fact, the majority of women don't develop heart disease until after age forty-five. Only one in one thousand women from age thirty-five to forty-four develops heart disease. The number rises to four per one thousand among women ages forty-five through fifty-four. By age seventy, the number of women with heart disease equals the number of men with the condition.

The increased risk with advancing age can partly be explained by the aging process itself. The connective tissues in the artery walls become stiffer and less flexible with age, a condition known as "hardening of the arteries," or *arteriosclerosis*. This may cause blood pressure to rise and may increase the heart's workload, causing the heart muscle itself to thicken and stiffen over time. Blood pressure and cholesterol levels tend to rise with age, too, which contributes to the increased risk.

Older women are also more likely to be diabetic, to be overweight, and to exercise less than younger women, all of which increase the risk (see below). In addition, after menopause, women lose the protective effect that estrogen provides.

Because of these age-related changes in the body, and because of the greater incidence of coronary artery disease among older women, the National Cholesterol Education Program now considers age to be a major coronary risk factor. *All* women over age fifty-five should consider themselves at risk.

Your Gender

Although coronary artery disease is the leading cause of death and disability for both men and women, men are more likely to succumb to heart disease at an earlier age than women, making younger men more vulnerable than younger women. Older women, however, are just as susceptible to heart disease as older men. What's more, some younger women—those with diabetes and certain hereditary forms of high blood cholesterol, for example—are just as vulnerable as younger men.

Your Cholesterol and Blood Lipid Levels

High cholesterol levels are associated with an increased risk of heart attack. People with total cholesterol levels of 240 milligrams per deciliter of blood (mg/dl) have more than twice the risk of people whose cholesterol is 200 mg/dl (see Table 3 on page 50). *Conversely, in people with high blood cholesterol (greater than 200 mg/dl), every 1 percent decline in total cholesterol is equivalent to a 2 percent decrease in risk.*

But total cholesterol levels tell only part of the story. In fact, it is possible to have total cholesterol levels in the "desirable" range (below 200 mg/dl) and still be at risk. For this reason, you and your doctor will also want to know your blood levels of LDL and HDL cholesterol and triglycerides, particularly if you have other risk factors for coronary artery disease.

If your LDL cholesterol is 130 or above, you are considered to be at a greater risk. Researchers are less certain about what levels of HDL cholesterol are associated with greater risk. In the major studies conducted to date, a range of HDL cholesterol levels have been associated with either an increased or decreased risk of heart disease. A 1992 National Institutes of Health Consensus Conference on Triglycerides and HDL Cholesterol

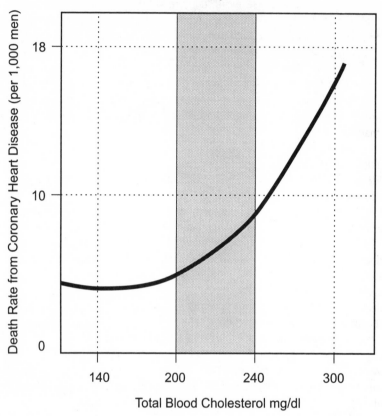

TABLE 3 — Blood Cholesterol Levels
and Your Risk of Coronary Heart Disease

As blood cholesterol levels rise, so does your risk of developing coronary heart disease.

arbitrarily chose levels less than 35 mg/dl of HDL cholesterol to indicate high risk. But the panel concedes that this may be too low for women.

For women, triglycerides are important, too, especially when high triglycerides team up with low levels of HDL cholesterol. The same NIH panel determined that a fasting triglyceride level of 500 mg/dl or more is considered "high" and a fasting triglyceride level between 250 and 500 mg/dl is "borderline high." We like to err on the side of conservatism, however. In our clinic, fasting triglyceride levels between 140 and 190 mg/dl are considered "above normal" and should be closely monitored. A fasting triglyceride level above 190 mg/dl is considered "high."

If your blood lipid levels indicate that you are at high risk, there are plenty of things you can do to improve your lipid profile and reduce your risk. These include eating a low-fat, low-cholesterol diet, exercising regularly, taking hormones if you are past menopause, and, if these measures don't work, taking one of a number of lipid-lowering drugs. You'll find more in-depth discussions about these protective measures in the chapters to come.

Your Blood Pressure

Elevated blood pressure is one of the most powerful contributors to the development of coronary artery disease. It is also a major cause of stroke. Even mildly elevated blood pressure leads to a greater incidence of atherosclerosis, heart attacks, and strokes.

Conversely, one of the most effective ways to prevent coronary artery disease is to keep your blood pressure in check. In fact, one of the largest studies to date, involving some 37,000 people, found that for every five to six points that a person's blood pressure is reduced, the risk of heart disease declines by 20 to 25 percent, and the risk of stroke by 30 to 40 percent. (For more on hypertension and how to manage it, see Chapter 13.)

Cigarette Smoking

We typically associate cigarette smoking with the development of lung cancer. But coronary artery disease is the largest smoking-related cause of death. *Nearly three times more smokers die of heart disease then lung cancer.* According to the American Heart Association, smokers are two times more likely to have a heart attack than nonsmokers. Moreover, smokers who have a heart attack are more likely to die within an hour than nonsmokers. Women who smoke and take birth control pills are up to thirty-nine times more likely to have a heart attack than women who don't smoke.

The risk of stroke—both from blood clots and cerebral hemorrhage—is doubled among women who smoke; heavy smokers (more than twenty-five cigarettes per day) have six times the risk of suffering a stroke than nonsmokers.

Cigarette smoking also increases the risk of nonsmoking family members who breathe in secondhand smoke. According to the American Heart

51 •

Association, "the risk of death due to heart disease is increased by about 30 percent among those exposed to environmental tobacco smoke at home." The risk could be much higher for those exposed at the workplace in which smoking is permitted, since more smokers contribute to greater levels of cigarette smoke in the air.

The good news is that smokers who quit reduce their risk of developing heart disease, regardless of how long or how much they have smoked. (For more on quitting, see Chapter 8.)

Your Exercise Habits

Sedentary living is now considered a major risk factor for heart disease, along with high blood pressure, high blood cholesterol, and cigarette smoking. Numerous studies have documented that inactive people are more likely to die of a heart attack than physically active people. A University of North Carolina study found, for instance, that sedentary women were three times more likely to die prematurely from heart attacks than physically active people. A program of regular moderate exercise can substantially reduce your risk (see Chapter 7).

Your Genes

As surprising as it sounds, coronary artery disease may well be one of the most common hereditary illnesses. Actually, it is not coronary artery disease itself that is inherited, but some of the main underlying causes of CAD—high blood lipids, hypertension, diabetes, obesity.

At least three major forms of high blood cholesterol appear to have genetic links. These include the following:

FAMILIAL HYPERCHOLESTEROLEMIA. About one in five hundred people is affected with this genetic disorder, making it the most common simple hereditary illness of all. People with familial hypercholesterolemia (FH) have a flaw in the gene that controls the production of *LDL receptors*. These receptors are specialized parts of the cell surface that attract and bind LDL cholesterol to the cell so it can be deposited there. People with FH are less efficient at clearing cholesterol from the bloodstream, or, in rare cases, are unable to do so at all. As a result, high levels of LDL cholesterol, VLDL cholesterol, and small-molecule LDL cholesterol build up in the bloodstream. Diets low in saturated fat and cholesterol and cholesterol-lowering drugs are often required to keep LDL cholesterol levels down.

TYPE III HYPERLIPOPROTEINEMIA. People with this genetic disorder usually have *low* levels of LDL cholesterol. However, a flaw in the gene that codes for apolipoprotein E causes these people to have high triglycerides and high levels of beta-VLDL cholesterol circulating in their bloodstream. Usually, though, the genetic defect is triggered by other medical conditions that can be controlled, including obesity, hypothyroidism, and diabetes.

FAMILIAL DEFECTIVE APO B-100. This newly discovered genetic abnormality is believed to be caused by a defect in the gene coding for apolipoprotein B. The genetic defect somehow keeps LDL cholesterol in the bloodstream from binding to LDL receptors in the body's cells resulting in dangerously high blood levels of LDL cholesterol. A few preliminary studies now suggest that as many as one in 500 people have this disorder, which would make it as common as familial hypercholesterolemia.

Having a family history of premature heart disease may be a sign that you are at risk of heart disease yourself, as Linda's story illustrates.

Case Report: Linda

Linda's father died of a heart attack when he was fifty-one. Her older brother had his first heart attack when he was just thirty-eight years old, and had had coronary bypass surgery by the time he was forty-one.

Linda thought she was immune from heart disease because she was a young woman. But at age thirty-nine, Linda developed severe chest pains and shortness of breath. Fortunately, she recognized these two classic signs of heart trouble and sought emergency medical help. An angiogram (an X-ray picture of the coronary arteries) revealed that one of Linda's coronary arteries was 90 percent blocked. The blockage was successfully treated, and Linda is doing fine now, determined to do what she can to prevent any further problems.

Like Linda, you may be at a greater risk if your father or a brother was diagnosed with or died of heart disease before age fifty-five, or if your mother or a sister developed heart disease before age sixty. You may also be at risk if your parents, brothers, or sisters have elevated cholesterol or triglyceride levels.

If you have a family history of high blood pressure or diabetes, you should consider yourself at risk as well. In fact, researchers strongly suspect that both of these conditions have genetic roots, too, although no one has been able to pinpoint a single genetic flaw leading to these medical conditions. It is likely that more than one gene is involved.

Keep in mind that what you inherit is not the disease itself, but a genetic predisposition to these medical conditions that can be influenced in numerous ways—many of which are within your control, such as your diet and exercise habits. So one of the most prevalent hereditary illnesses may also be one of the most preventable.

Contributing Risk Factors

The following risk factors are known to contribute to an increased risk of heart disease, but the extent to which they do so is still under investigation.

Early Menopause

Postmenopausal women are more than twice as likely to develop heart disease as premenopausal women. This is believed to be due largely to the dramatic drop in estrogen produced by the ovaries at the time of menopause.

Women who have an early natural menopause—that is, whose menopause occurs before age forty-five—have a somewhat greater risk of developing coronary artery disease than women whose menopause occurs later (age fifty or older). This is simply because these women lose the protection afforded by estrogen that much earlier than women whose menopause occurs later in life. In one Boston University study, women whose menopause occurred before age forty-five (and who did not take estrogen) were estimated to have a 60 percent greater risk of heart attack than women whose menopause occurred after age fifty. Those whose menopause occurred between ages forty-five and forty-nine had a 20 percent higher risk than the over-fifty group.

Postmenopausal estrogen preparations can help reduce the risk, as can such lifestyle measures as eating a low-fat diet, exercising regularly, and not smoking.

Previous Hysterectomy or Ovariectomy

Women who have their ovaries surgically removed before a natural menopause undergo an instantaneous "surgical" menopause. Because they lose their main source of estrogen—the ovaries—these women are at a much greater risk of developing heart disease than women whose ovaries remain intact and functional until the time of a natural menopause. The younger a woman is when she has the surgery, the greater is her risk. One study reported that the risk of heart attack was 7.2 times higher for women whose ovaries were removed before age thirty-five, compared with women who had not had the operation.

What about premenopausal women who have had a hysterectomy (surgical removal of the uterus) but whose ovaries remain intact? Technically, these women are not considered menopausal, since the ovaries continue to produce estrogen and progesterone until a natural menopause occurs. Some studies have found only a slightly increased risk of heart disease among women who have had a hysterectomy. But others have found that even these women are at an increased risk of developing heart disease. The Framingham Heart Study, for instance, reported that removal of either the uterus alone, or removal of both the uterus and one or both ovaries increases a woman's risk of coronary artery disease.

How could surgical removal of the uterus increase a woman's risk of developing heart disease? Some studies have suggested that ovaries left intact after a hysterectomy may not function as well as they did before the uterus was removed because of impaired blood flow to the ovaries. What's more, research has suggested that up to one-third of all women who have a hysterectomy may experience an early menopause as a result of ovarian failure. The low estrogen levels associated with poorly functioning or nonfunctioning ovaries after a hysterectomy could help explain the increased risk of heart disease that some research has associated with this operation.

If you have had both ovaries removed during your reproductive years, you are definitely at increased risk of developing heart disease and should consider using estrogen in addition to other protective measures. If you have had a hysterectomy in your premenopausal years and your ovaries were left intact, you should annually have a blood test for follicle-stimulating hormone (FSH), which can help determine whether or not your ovaries are still producing adequate levels of protective estrogen. If FSH levels begin to rise or if you begin developing other symptoms of menopause, such as hot flashes, you should plan accordingly with such risk-reducing strategies as adopting a low-fat diet and regular exercise. You may also want to consider using postmenopausal estrogen preparations.

Diabetes

Diabetes mellitus is particularly hard on women. Several studies have confirmed that the condition somehow completely wipes out the biological protection against heart disease that healthy women enjoy. In fact, some studies have demonstrated that women with diabetes are at a greater risk of developing coronary artery disease than men with diabetes.

Diabetes is a disorder related to your body's ability to use or *metabolize* the energy from the food you eat. It is caused by either a deficiency of or an impairment in the action of *insulin*, a hormone secreted by the pancreas gland located just behind the stomach. Insulin helps your body's tissues store and use the sugars (glucose), protein, and fats circulating in your bloodstream after a meal. There are two types of diabetes: insulin-dependent diabetes, which typically develops during childhood or early adulthood and requires daily insulin injections, and non-insulin-dependent diabetes, which usually doesn't develop until the middle years. For reasons that aren't clear, about two-thirds more women than men develop non-insulin-dependent diabetes.

Both types of diabetes dramatically increase the risk of developing coronary artery disease in men and women. In fact, more than 80 percent of people with diabetes die of some form of heart or blood vessel disease. Both men and women with diabetes tend to develop atherosclerosis at an earlier age than those who don't have diabetes, and the blockage tends to be more severe.

Heart disease is just one of several major complications associated with diabetes, including kidney failure, amputations due to infection, and blindness. Better control of diabetes is associated with fewer complications. And the majority of women with non-insulin-dependent diabetes can control it with dietary changes alone. For more on diabetes, see Chapter 8.)

As mentioned earlier, even if you *don't* now have diabetes, having a family history of the disorder increases your risk of developing coronary artery disease. And since non-insulin-dependent diabetes can go undetected for many years, if you are over age forty with a family history of diabetes, or if you have had a baby weighing more than nine pounds at birth, you should undergo an annual screening test for diabetes.

Your Weight

Being overweight (more than 30 percent over your "desirable" or "ideal" weight) increases your risk of developing heart disease even if you have no other risk factors. In a study by JoAnn Manson, M.D., and her colleagues at Harvard University, even mildly overweight women were up to forty times more likely to develop coronary artery disease than normal-weight women. And women who gained weight *during the middle years* had double the risk of developing coronary artery disease than women who had been overweight all their lives. More recently, Walter C. Willett, M.D., and colleagues at

Harvard University's Division of Preventive Medicine, reported that even higher body weights within the "normal" range, as well as modest weight gains after age eighteen, also are associated with an increased risk of coronary heart disease in middle-aged women. These findings are particularly alarming because they suggest that the current weight guidelines issued by the U.S. Department of Agriculture in 1990—weight guidelines that suggest you can maintain good health while weighing a little more than earlier weight tables—might give false reassurances to the large number of women in this country over age thirty-five whose weight falls within the "normal" range of current guidelines.

Women who tend to put on weight around the waist and abdomen ("apple" body shapes) appear to be most at risk. These women are more likely to have lower levels of HDL cholesterol, elevated LDL cholesterol, triglycerides, and insulin, and are more likely to develop hypertension and diabetes than women who accumulate fat around the buttocks and thighs ("pear" body shapes). (For more on determining the distribution of body fat, see page 65.)

Excess weight increases the strain on the heart. Obesity also increases blood pressure and blood lipid levels, and increases your risk of developing non-insulin-dependent diabetes.

Dr. Manson estimates that *as much as 40 percent of coronary disease in women could be prevented by weight loss alone.* Losing weight is often enough to lower elevated blood cholesterol and blood pressure and to keep non-insulin-dependent diabetes in check without drugs and their sometimes serious side effects.

Ethnic Background

For reasons that aren't clear, black women are 24 percent more likely to die of coronary heart disease than white women. Black women also generally experience their first heart attack about five years earlier than white women, and, after suffering a heart attack, are less likely to survive than whites.

This excess risk for coronary heart disease can be directly traced to genetic differences, lifestyle factors, and economic disadvantage. For instance, black women are more likely to develop hypertension (a major risk factor for coronary artery disease) than white women, and at an earlier age than white women. Researchers suspect that this increased susceptibility to hypertension is caused, in part, by genetic differences between the two races.

African-American women are also more prone to develop weight problems, which are associated with an increased risk of heart disease. Among twenty- to thirty-two-year-old adult women, 24 percent of black women are obese, compared with only 11 percent of white women.

Studies have found that, overall, African-Americans smoke cigarettes more than Caucasians, which also increases their risk.

Inadequate access to preventive health care and economic disadvantage also play a role in the premature development of heart problems among black women, and in the poorer prognosis for them.

If you are a black woman, you should consider yourself at increased risk of developing heart problems—especially hypertension. You will need to take a good hard look at any other modifiable risk factors you have, and make an extra effort to do what you can to lower your risk.

Other Possible Risk Factors

The following may also influence your risk of heart disease, although more research needs to be conducted before their exact role in the development of heart disease is known.

Emotional Stress

There is general concern that women today—particularly those who work outside the home—are subjected to more stress than in the past, and that the added stress may adversely influence their risk of coronary artery disease. How so? Emotional stress triggers a physiological reaction in the body known as the "fight-or-flight response," in which the adrenal glands pump out a flood of hormones, notably *epinephrine* and *norepinephrine*. These hormones accelerate your breathing and heart rate, raise your blood pressure and blood sugar levels, and release high-energy fats into the bloodstream for quick energy, essentially preparing you for a fight with or a quick flight away from a physical threat. The hormones also increase the stickiness of blood platelets, which makes blood clot more easily (in case you're wounded in the ensuing battle). *Cortisol*, another hormone released from the adrenal glands when your body is chronically stressed, raises blood cholesterol levels.

Several studies have suggested that the constant firing of the fight-or-flight response from living in a stressful environment may lead to permanent increases in heart rate, blood pressure, and, possibly, blood cholesterol levels, all of which increase the risk of developing heart disease.

So far, few major studies have been conducted on the effects of stress on a woman's risk of developing heart disease. Interestingly, most of the studies conducted to date have found overall that women in the workplace have *fewer* risk factors for heart disease than homemakers, including higher levels of HDL cholesterol, lower levels of triglycerides and blood cholesterol, and lower blood pressure. Moreover, working women in the studies were more likely to exercise and less likely to smoke than homemakers.

There is, however, some evidence to suggest that the type of work you do outside of the home may influence your risk. Women in occupations that involve a lot of responsibility but little control, such as nursing and clerical jobs, may be at a greater risk of developing cardiovascular disease. But again, the studies conducted so far have not consistently found this to be true.

Other studies have suggested that the multiple roles women assume today—juggling work and family roles simultaneously—may be associated with an increased risk of heart disease. In the Framingham Heart Study, for example, the eight-year incidence of heart disease increased among women working outside of the home as the number of children increased. And as we mentioned in Chapter 1, Swedish researchers found that women continue to exhibit increased cardiovascular arousal after returning home from work in the evening, rather than unwinding, as men do. Still, no research has linked multiple roles or stress with an increased risk of death from cardiovascular disease among women.

What about the so-called coronary-prone or Type A personality? Studies have found a strong correlation between a cluster of personality traits, including competitiveness, aggression, hostility, impatience, and time urgency, and an increased risk of heart attacks *in men*. But few studies have been conducted on women, so the issue remains controversial. One study found that women who suppressed their anger were more likely to die of heart disease, cancer, and numerous other causes of death. The Framingham Heart Study also found that working women who did not discuss their anger were more likely to have angina than women who did express their anger. The findings didn't carry over to homemakers in the study, however.

Fourteen- and twenty-year follow-up studies on women participating in the Framingham study found that those with Type A personality traits were also more likely to develop angina.

Still other research has linked anxiety and depression with an increased risk of angina. And in an eight-year study, the Framingham researchers found the incidence of heart disease was much higher among women with both Type A behavior *and* symptoms of depression.

Many questions remain unanswered about the role of stress and heart disease in women, but the evidence so far is convincing enough that you should not ignore stress as a possible risk factor for heart disease.

Iron

As a woman, you're probably used to worrying about getting enough iron to ward off iron-deficiency anemia. In fact, throughout your reproductive years, you lose iron every time you menstruate, which tends to keep your body's iron stores (the backup supply of iron tucked away in muscle and other tissues) low. Once you stop menstruating, however, your body's iron stores rise quickly (see Table 4). According to a 1992 report from Finnish researchers, therein lies the problem. The Finnish scientists found that the level of stored iron *in men* is a strong risk factor for heart disease— possibly stronger than the risk factors of elevated blood cholesterol, high blood pressure, or diabetes. In the five-year study involving 1,931 men, even "normal" levels of stored iron were strongly associated with an increased risk of heart attack, and every 1 percent increase in serum ferritin (storage iron) was associated with a more than 4 percent increase in the risk of heart attack. A high ferritin level—200 micrograms or more per liter of blood—more than doubled the relative risk of a heart attack. If further research confirms these results, the iron theory could help explain why women appear to be safe from heart attacks until after menopause, when iron stores accumulate quite rapidly.

How can high levels of storage iron contribute to heart disease? The researchers point out that the release of iron from ferritin molecules may contribute to the formation of oxygen free radicals, which could help transform LDL cholesterol into an oxidized form that more readily adheres to and clogs artery walls. The ferritin molecules are also capable of releasing iron at the site of tissue damage, which could help cause the injury to the heart muscle that follows a heart attack. Some animal experiments have suggested that iron depletion may inhibit both the clogging of the arteries that leads to a heart attack and the injury to the heart muscle after a heart attack. The iron theory could also help explain the protective effects of aspirin, fish oils, and a cholesterol-lowering drug called cholestyramine. Aspirin and fish oils increase the time it takes your blood to clot, which may increase chronic blood loss and therefore lower iron stores in the body. Cholestyramine, which passes through the body without being absorbed, has been used to make animals iron-deficient.

A few subsequent studies have failed to find an association between high levels of ferritin and increased risk of heart disease. But most of the studies were small, and may not carry as much weight as the Finnish study. The largest study to find no association between storage iron and

TABLE 4 — Pre- and Postmenopausal Levels of Storage Iron

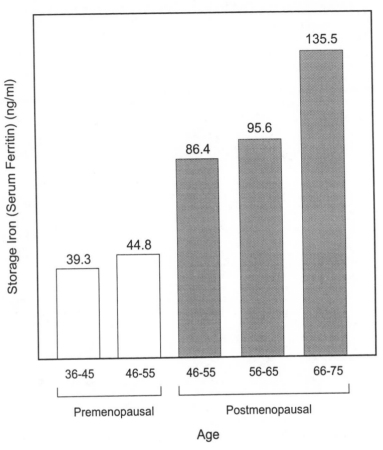

heart disease involved some 46,932 patients at the Kaiser Permanente Medical Care Program in Oakland, California. The researchers in that study measured the patients' *transferrin saturation level* (TS), rather than serum ferritin, and found only a marginally increased risk of heart attack among those whose TS levels were high.

The bottom line is that it is still not clear what role ferritin plays in the development of heart disease. So if you are past menopause, don't stop eating iron-rich foods just yet.

Fibrinogen

High levels of this blood coagulant have been associated with an increased risk of coronary artery disease in men. Exercise reduces blood levels of fibrinogen, which may be one way in which regular physical activity helps protect against heart disease.

Male/Female Pattern Baldness

Male/female pattern baldness is a hereditary type of hair loss triggered by high levels of the "male" hormone androgen. Although the condition is much more common among men, some women are affected, too. Unlike men, who develop an M-shaped hairline with thinning in the temporal areas, thinning of hair in women occurs in a more diffuse pattern. Some women with this condition may also develop an uncharacteristic overgrowth of facial hair, deepening of the voice, increased muscle mass, and other signs of masculinization.

At least one recent study has associated pattern baldness with a modest increase in risk of heart disease in men. No research has been conducted on women with the condition. Until further studies are completed, however, it would be prudent for women with pattern baldness to heed the advice for men with the condition: follow a heart-healthy lifestyle that includes a low-fat diet, regular exercise, and other protective measures described in the chapters ahead.

Cocaine Abuse

Preliminary studies on young people who died from cocaine abuse have suggested that use of cocaine may hasten the development of atherosclerotic lesions in the arteries. In a preliminary report, Renu Virmani, M.D., chairman of cardiovascular pathology at the Armed Forces Institute of Pathology in Washington, studied thirty-nine patients with an average age of twenty-five, twenty of whom were known to be habitual cocaine abusers.

Virmani found little difference in the amounts of total cholesterol or HDL cholesterol between the cocaine abusers and a group of nineteen young accident victims who had not used cocaine. But she did find more plaque buildup in the arteries of people who had been using cocaine than in those who had not been using the drug. The scientists speculate that cocaine may promote plaque buildup in many ways: by causing inflammation of the arteries, by temporarily increasing blood pressure, and by increasing the permeability of the endothelium (lining of the blood vessel walls), allowing fat to pass more easily through the endothelium.

B-Vitamin Deficiencies

Years ago, researchers noted that children with a rare genetic disease, *homocystinuria*, accumulated extremely high circulating levels of the amino acid *homocysteine* as a result of an enzyme deficiency. These children usually died of cardiovascular disease at a young age. Scientists knew even then that homocysteine was necessary for the production of two other amino acids, *cysteine* and *methionine*. They also knew that the B vitamins folate, B_6, and B_{12} were a crucial part of the body's production of these two amino acids. The question arose: Would high levels of homocysteine resulting from a low intake of folate, B_6, or B_{12} increase an adult's risk of premature heart disease?

Recent studies suggest that this is so. Researchers from England and Ireland found in 1991 that 28 to 42 percent of patients with cardiovascular disease had elevated levels of homocysteine. They concluded that people with high blood levels of homocysteine were nearly twenty-eight times more likely to develop premature vascular disease than those with normal levels. More recent studies support the findings of the British and Irish researchers.

Then came a report from the Framingham Heart Study showing that low intakes of folate, B_6, and B_{12} were, in fact, associated with higher levels of homocysteine. Of the 1,100 Framingham residents who participated in the study, 30 percent had high levels of homocysteine. And two-thirds of these people had levels of these vitamins below the Recommended Dietary Allowance (RDA).

While it is not known exactly how homocysteine contributes to heart disease, high blood levels of homocysteine are thought to reduce the production of nitric oxide by the blood vessel wall, possibly causing the blood vessel to become constricted. Homocysteine may also interfere with the activation of protein C, a natural anticoagulant, thus helping to encourage the development of blood clots.

Having one or two risk factors for coronary artery disease doesn't mean that you definitely will develop heart trouble in the future. But it does indicate that your chances of developing heart disease are somewhat greater than those of people without any risk factors. Having one or more risk factors is also an indication that you should routinely undergo certain basic cardiovascular screening tests, the topic of the next chapter.

CHAPTER 5

Common Screening and Diagnostic Tests

REGARDLESS OF WHETHER you have any of the risk factors discussed in Chapter 4, you should periodically undergo certain basic screening tests for coronary artery disease. If the screening tests reveal a problem, or if you already have one or more risk factors for heart disease, you should consider having a more formal cardiovascular workup. If your doctor doesn't recommend it, *you* should demand it.

In the pages that follow, you'll learn about some of the basic screening tests that may be offered, as well as some of the more advanced tests used to diagnose existing coronary artery disease.

Basic Screening Tests for Coronary Artery Disease

A cardiovascular evaluation should begin with a few basic screening tests. These include the following:

Weight

Overweight women are at a greater risk of developing heart disease than women of normal weight. So weighing in at the doctor's office will be an important first step in your cardiovascular evaluation. To help you determine your "desirable" weight, see the 1983 Metropolitan Life Insurance Company's standardized height and weight tables on page 286.

Weighing yourself on a conventional scale is a start, but there's a lot the scales don't tell you. For instance, you can be overfat without being overweight; that is, you can have a high percentage of body fat and still register normal weight on the scales. This is why it is important to know your percentage of body fat as well as your weight. There are a number of ways to do this. One of the easiest is to calculate your *body-mass index* (BMI). To determine your body-mass index, find your present weight in the left-hand column of the table on pages 284–285. Then read across to the column with your height.

Another way to estimate your percentage of body fat is by having your doctor or other qualified health professional perform a *skin-fold test*. The concept is based on the fact that about half of your total body fat is in the tissues just under the skin. Skin-fold calipers are used to gently pull the skin and fat away from the muscle and measure its thickness.

More advanced—and more accurate—means of determining your percentage of body fat are slowly becoming available. Ask your doctor for more information.

Perhaps more important than *how much* fat you have is *where* fat accumulates on your body. Remember: Women with apple-shaped bodies, in which fat accumulates around the waist, are more likely to have high levels of LDL cholesterol, low levels of HDL cholesterol, high insulin levels, and high blood pressure than women with pear-shaped bodies, in which fat accumulates around the buttocks and upper thighs.

One of the best ways to determine *where* fat is accumulating on your body is by measuring your waist-to-hip ratio. Recent studies have found the waist-to-hip ratio to be *one of the most accurate* weight-related gauges of a woman's risk of developing heart disease (as well as a host of other obesity-related conditions, such as breast and endometrial cancer and gallbladder disease). In a recent study investigating body fat distribution and risk of death in older women, the higher the waist-to-hip ratio, the greater the risk of dying of an obesity-related medical problem (including heart disease) during the five-year study. Women most at risk had a *high* waist-to-hip ratio and a *low* body mass index.

To determine your waist-to-hip ratio, use a cloth measuring tape to measure your waist about an inch above your navel. Measure your hips at the widest point between your hips and your buttocks. Now divide your waist measurement by your hip measurement. (For example, if your waist measurement is 32 and your hip measurement is 36, your waist-to-hip ratio would be calculated in this way: 32 ÷ 36 = 0.89). A waist-to-hip ratio greater than 0.80 for women signals greater health risks.

Blood Pressure

Since hypertension is one of the major risk factors for coronary artery disease, you should have your blood pressure checked at least once a year. Because hypertension is virtually symptomless and can go undetected for years, most physicians now regularly check your blood pressure every time you visit.

Your doctor will check your blood pressure by wrapping an inflatable cuff around your upper arm, tightening the cuff until blood flow in your arm is temporarily cut off, then listening through, a stethoscope as the cuff is loosened and blood flow is restored. A blood pressure reading consists of two numbers written as a fraction: the top number (*systolic* pressure) represents the force of blood on the arteries as the heart contracts; the bottom number (*diastolic* pressure) is blood pressure when the heart is at rest. A reading of 130/85 or lower is considered normal. (For more on the diagnosis and treatment of hypertension, see Chapter 13.)

Ankle/Arm Blood Pressure Index (AAI)

Although a blood pressure reading usually involves having a blood pressure cuff wrapped around your arm, don't be surprised if your doctor also takes a blood pressure reading from your ankle as well. Recent studies have found that the ratio of systolic blood pressure (the top number of a blood pressure reading) from your ankle and arm, known as the ankle/arm blood pressure index, or AAI, is a quick and easy way to predict increased heart disease risk, especially in women over age sixty-five. The test is used to determine whether or not you have artery disease in the legs, a condition known as *peripheral arterial disease*, or PAD. Peripheral arterial disease of the legs has been associated with an increased risk for heart attacks and strokes. In one study involving 5,200 older adults from four communities across the country, those with a low ankle/arm index were two to three times more likely to die within a few years than were those without any evidence of hidden (or subclinical) arterial disease. And in a 1993 study of nearly 1,500 women age sixty-five and older, the ankle/arm blood pressure index was a better predictor of increased risk than blood cholesterol levels.

If you have a low AAI (0.9 or less), you may be a candidate for aggressive therapy to lower your risk of heart disease, even if you have none of the traditional risk factors for heart disease, such as high blood cholesterol, or if you have no obvious signs of existing heart disease, such as chest pains.

Cholesterol and Blood Lipid Tests

The National Cholesterol Education Program recommends that all adults age twenty or older have their total blood cholesterol level measured once every five years. You may have already had a simple screening test that measures total cholesterol from a drop of blood, and that's a start. We feel, however, that this test is not comprehensive enough to evaluate your risk of developing heart disease, especially if you have one or more of the risk factors described in Chapter 4. For a more accurate assessment of your risk, it is essential that you undergo a complete *lipid profile*, which will give you not only your total cholesterol levels, but also levels of triglycerides, HDL cholesterol, LDL cholesterol, and the ratio of total cholesterol to HDL cholesterol.

Linda's story illustrates the importance of having a lipid profile to help determine your risk rather than just a finger-prick test for total cholesterol. As you may recall from Chapter 4, Linda had a strong family history of heart disease; both her father and brother had developed heart problems before age fifty-five. When she came to our clinic at age thirty-two for treatment of a chronic vaginal infection, we advised her to have her cholesterol tested, as well, because of her family history. The lipid profile revealed that Linda's total cholesterol level was 143 mg/dl—in the "desirable" range. Based on total cholesterol alone, Linda did not appear to be at an increased risk of developing heart problems herself. But the lipid profile also found that Linda's triglycerides—391 mg/dl—were elevated, and her HDL cholesterol, at 30 mg/dl, was low. This combination of high triglycerides and low HDL cholesterol signaled an increased risk, in spite of her "normal" total cholesterol level.

Here is another example of how total cholesterol levels alone can be misleading. Sixty-six-year-old Sarah came to our clinic complaining of heart palpitations and other anxiety-related symptoms. Her total cholesterol, at 261 mg/dl, put her in the "high risk" category. But further testing revealed that Sarah's triglycerides, at 167 mg/dl, were low, and her HDL cholesterol was a healthy 94 mg/dl, pointing to a lower overall risk.

The lipid profile involves having blood drawn from a vein in your arm. Because the test results (mainly triglycerides) can be influenced by what you eat, you should have the test done after an overnight fast.

The lipid profile is important because it can often help uncover possible causes of high blood cholesterol, which will influence the type of treatment you receive. Some lipid profiles—high triglycerides and normal levels of LDL cholesterol, for example—suggest the cause may be genetic, particularly if other family members share the same lipid pattern. Under certain circumstances, you may need to take cholesterol-lowering drugs under the care of a cardiologist or lipid specialist. If your cholesterol levels rise only after menopause, the problem may simply be menopause-related, and hormone therapy may be appropriate.

We recommend that all women have a lipid profile at least once before menopause—even if your total cholesterol is in the "desirable" range. If your blood cholesterol levels are normal (see "Interpreting the Results of Your Cholesterol Test" on the next page), you should repeat the test once every five years until menopause. After menopause, you should have a lipid profile every one to two years to monitor any menopause-related changes.

If your cholesterol levels are elevated to begin with, your physician will probably want to test you more frequently—even as often as every six months—to see how well various lipid-lowering therapies (including diet and exercise) are working.

SHOULD CHILDREN AND ADOLESCENTS HAVE A CHOLESTEROL TEST?

At what age should you (or your children) begin having your cholesterol tested? This is not an easy question to answer. The problem is that mass screening tests for total cholesterol can sometimes be inaccurate; total cholesterol readings taken from the same person at about the same time (from a few hours to a few days apart) can vary by as much as 15 points. Moreover, children's cholesterol levels fluctuate quite a bit, and are influenced by diet, stress, exercise, puberty, and weight changes. At least one study has suggested that some children with high cholesterol may outgrow the condition. Because heart disease rarely develops before midlife, some experts have even questioned the wisdom of the National Cholesterol Education Program's recommendation that young adults in their twenties and thirties routinely have their cholesterol tested.

For these reasons, the American Heart Association, the American Academy of Pediatrics, and other health organizations decided against screening all children for elevated blood cholesterol. The groups do advocate screening for some children, however, and you should notify your pediatrician if your child is over age two and his or her parents, grandparents, uncles, or aunts had or have:

Should Children and Adolescents Have a Cholesterol Test? (Cont.)

- high cholesterol levels
- early cardiovascular disease (under age fifty-five for men or under age sixty for women)
- a history of sudden death or stroke
- other signs of heart disease, such as angina

Children should undergo repeated measurements before a diagnosis is made. Youngsters with cholesterol levels above 170 mg/dl should also have a lipid profile. Even if total blood cholesterol measurements are normal, at-risk children should have repeat cholesterol tests every two to three years.

If your child has high blood cholesterol levels or other risk factors for heart disease, *do not* attempt to treat it on your own. Some studies have shown that low-fat diets and other preventive measures that work well for adults do more harm than good in children, especially those under age two. Rather, you should plan to work closely with your pediatrician to manage your child's condition.

Interpreting the Results of Your Cholesterol Test

Total cholesterol

Below 200 mg/dl	Desirable
200 to 239 mg/dl	Borderline high risk
240 mg/dl or above	High risk

Low-density lipoproteins

Below 130 mg/dl	Desirable
130 to 159 mg/dl	Borderline high risk
160 mg/dl or above	High risk

High-density lipoproteins

Below 35 mg/dl	Increased risk
35 to 50 mg/dl	Good
50 mg/dl or above	Better

Triglycerides

20 to 140 mg/dl	Normal
140 to 190 mg/dl	Above normal—monitor
Above 190 mg/dl	High

Total cholesterol/HDL cholesterol

Below 4.5	Decreased risk
Above 4.5	Increased risk

Fasting Blood Glucose Test

Remember: Having diabetes increases your risk of developing cardiovascular problems. Diabetes often causes no symptoms—especially in its early stages—and can go undetected for years. For this reason, it is a good idea to have your blood sugar levels periodically tested after age forty-five.

Sometimes, rising blood sugar levels indicate an increased risk even when blood cholesterol levels are normal, as Christine's story illustrates. Christine came to our clinic at age fifty-seven seeking relief from hot flashes and other menopausal symptoms. Because she was menopausal and had hypertension, we recommended that she also have her blood cholesterol and blood sugar levels monitored. Her cholesterol levels were normal, but, over the years, her blood sugar level began to climb, from 96 mg/dl to 105 mg/dl and, at her last evaluation at age sixty-two, to 113 mg/dl. Her rising blood sugar levels coincided with a weight gain of seventeen pounds, which probably was contributing to increased insulin resistance, in which her body used insulin less efficiently. Christine's weight gain, together with her rising blood sugar levels, put her at increased risk of developing diabetes and heart trouble. Fortunately, the problem was caught in its earliest stages, and can probably be remedied with weight loss alone.

Your physician may recommend that you be screened for diabetes if you

- have a family history of diabetes
- are more than 20 percent over your desirable weight or have a waist-to-hip ratio above 0.80
- have given birth to a baby weighing more than nine pounds or have given birth to progressively larger babies
- have had gestational diabetes (diabetes that develops during pregnancy)
- have a history of recurrent skin, genital, or urinary tract infections
- are between the twenty-fourth and twenty-eighth weeks of pregnancy.
- have any of the signs or symptoms of diabetes, such as increased urination, increased thirst, or sugar in the urine

The *fasting blood glucose test* is often used to screen for diabetes. The test involves having blood drawn from your arm after an overnight fast so that laboratory technicians can test for blood sugar levels. Blood sugar levels below 115 mg/dl are considered normal. Fasting blood sugar levels that are 140 mg/dl or higher on at least two separate occasions indicate that you have diabetes. You may also be at increased risk of developing diabetes if you experience a progressive increase in fasting blood sugar levels that are within the normal range (below 115 mg/dl), as was the case with Christine.

If a fasting blood glucose test indicates that blood sugar levels are greater than 115 mg/dl but less than 140 mg/dl, or if you have a progressive increase in fasting blood sugar levels below 115 mg/dl, your doctor may recommend that you undergo a two-hour glucose-tolerance test. This test measures how the body responds to an increase in blood sugar over time. During the test, your blood sugar is measured before you consume a concentrated glucose drink, and again one and two hours later.

Uric Acid Test

Uric acid is a byproduct of metabolism and can be measured in blood and urine. Normally, uric acid measurement is used to screen for kidney disease and to detect certain metabolic disorders, such as gout. However, high blood levels of uric acid (*hyperuricemia*) have also been associated with hypertension, coronary artery disease, obesity, high blood lipid levels, diabetes, and toxemia of pregnancy. Some studies have documented a high uric acid level as being a risk factor for coronary artery disease.

To determine your blood level of uric acid, blood will be drawn from a vein in your arm and sent to a laboratory for analysis. Although there are no food or fluid restrictions prior to the test, blood uric acid levels can be influenced by certain foods. For this reason, during the day or two before the test, you may want to limit your intake of foods high in the amino acid *purine*, such as organ meats, scallops, sardines, anchovies, asparagus, mushrooms, and spinach.

Normal blood levels of uric acid are between 2.5 and 7.5 mg/dl.

In the Near Future

Eventually, a cardiovascular evaluation will include blood tests for apolipo-proteins, small-molecule LDL cholesterol, and other subgroups of choles-terol that will allow physicians to gauge your risk more accurately. Some of these tests are already being used for research purposes, but for now, the tests are too complicated and too costly to be of much practical value. A few tests are worth mentioning, however, because they are inexpensive, easy to perform, and, when used along with the current screening tests, soon may be able to give a more accurate picture of your risk.

Blood Homocysteine Levels

A blood test that measures levels of the amino acid homocysteine may be helpful in predicting people at high risk of developing heart disease. Some twenty scientific studies involving more than two thousand patients have consistently found that people who have had a stroke or some other form of cardiovascular disease tend to have higher blood levels of homocysteine than those with no cardiovascular disease.

Triglyceride-Tolerance Test

Although blood tests that measure triglycerides are conducted while you are fasting, some experts have suggested that a better approach might be to determine how the body processes triglycerides over time. This would involve testing triglyceride levels periodically (once every hour or two) after you have ingested a high-fat meal.

Common Diagnostic Tests

If you are over age fifty-five and have one or more risk factors for coronary artery disease, or if screening tests suggest that you have a problem, additional diagnostic tests may be in order. The following tests are also routinely used to evaluate the causes of any chest pain you may have.

Resting Electrocardiogram (ECG)

This test is used to monitor the electrical activity of the heart. The test can help determine whether you have previously had a heart attack that you were unaware of (silent myocardial infarction); left ventricular hypertrophy (enlargement of the heart); arrhythmias (abnormal heart rhythms); or a blockage in one or more of the coronary arteries.

Your doctor may recommend that you have an ECG if you have any of the risk factors for coronary artery disease along with symptoms of heart disease, such as shortness of breath, chest pain, dizziness, palpitations, or fainting. An ECG is sometimes offered as part of a routine physical if you are over forty.

The test is painless, noninvasive, and takes less than fifteen minutes. During the test, your doctor or other qualified health professional will place numerous electrodes (also called leads) at various positions on the body. Once the electrodes are in place, you simply sit or lie quietly while a machine records on graph paper the electrical impulses generated by your heart.

The biggest drawback to the ECG is that it has limited usefulness as a screening test. For example, a normal ECG does not necessarily mean that you *do not* have coronary artery disease. ECG changes often do not become apparent until narrowing of the arteries has become severe enough to cause a serious disruption of blood flow.

On the other hand, an abnormal ECG does not provide conclusive evidence that you *do* have coronary artery disease, especially if you have no symptoms and no risk factors for heart disease. For this reason, your doctor will probably order further diagnostic tests if you have an abnormal ECG.

Exercise Stress Test
The purpose of the exercise stress test (also known as a "stress test") is to determine how well the heart functions under physical stress, and to check for arrhythmias, narrowing of the coronary arteries, and *ischemia* (reduced blood flow to the heart muscle, usually caused by atherosclerosis). One of the main reasons for having a stress test at our clinic is to determine your level of physical fitness, your muscle strength and endurance, and your maximum heart rate, all of which can be used to develop an exercise program suited to your needs (see Chapter 7).

The only difference between the stress test and the resting ECG is that during the exercise stress test, the ECG monitors your heart's electrical activity while you exercise on a treadmill or stationary bicycle. The reasoning behind the test is simple: coronary arteries that are blocked may function adequately while you are at rest, but during physical exertion they may not be able to meet the heart's increased need for oxygen. This causes characteristic changes in the heart's electrical activity, which can be read on an ECG.

If you are over fifty-five and have one or more risk factors for coronary artery disease, or if you already have signs of coronary artery disease, such as chest pains, you may be advised to have an exercise stress test. The test is also recommended for sedentary men and women over age forty-five who wish to begin an exercise program.

During the test, a blood pressure cuff is wrapped around your arm and several electrodes are attached to your chest. Your heart's electrical activity, heart rate, and blood pressure are measured while you are at rest; you then begin to exercise on a treadmill or stationary bicycle. The speed and or the angle of the treadmill or the resistance of the bicycle is gradually increased to increase the heart's workload. The test will be stopped immediately if your doctor detects any abnormal heart rhythms, or if you report chest pains, dizziness, shortness of breath, or other serious signs of distress. Be sure to tell your doctor if you have any of these symptoms while the test is in progress. If not, the bicycle test continues for a set period of time (usually six minutes), and the treadmill test continues until you are too tired to continue. Your heart's rate and rhythm and blood pressure will continue to be monitored for five to fifteen minutes after the test, while you recover.

Like the ECG, the exercise stress test is not perfect. Several studies have reported high rates of "false-positive" results among healthy, symptom-free women who have an exercise stress test. Depending on which study you look at, false-positive test results have varied from 32 to 67 percent, which some experts say is unacceptably high.

Why is the rate of false-positive results so high among women? Some researchers believe that different methods of testing and interpretation of the results may explain some of the false-positive tests. Others point out that older women who have an exercise stress test are more likely to be out of shape or to have medical conditions other than heart disease, both of which may keep them from excerising strenuously enough for the results to be valid. Other heart conditions, such as mitral valve prolapse, spasms of the coronary arteries, and certain drugs also may influence the test results.

Because of the high rate of false-positive results among women, you and your doctor should keep in mind that an abnormal stress test doesn't necessarily mean that you have coronary artery disease. But if you finish the test with a *negative* result, you can rest assured that you probably *don't* have coronary artery disease. The test is more accurate in its ability to rule out coronary artery disease than to diagnose it.

Thallium Exercise Stress Test

If you have an abnormal resting ECG, your doctor may recommend that you have a thallium exercise stress test. The test is identical to the exercise stress with one exception: at the peak of exercise, or immediately after exercise, a small amount of the radioactive material *thallium* is injected into a vein in your arm. After you stop exercising, you will be sent to a nuclear medicine imaging camera, which will scan your heart for the next twenty minutes, and measure the number of gamma rays given off by the

FIGURE 6 — Thallium Scan for Thallium Stress Test

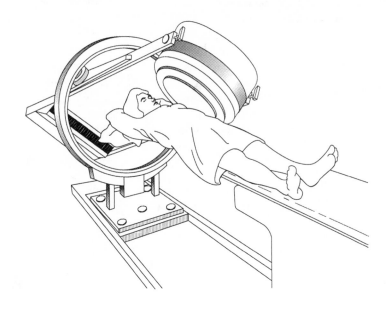

thallium (see Figure 6 above). The thallium scan is repeated several hours later or the following day, while you are at rest, and the results of both scans are compared. A decrease in the amount of gamma rays immediately after the exercise test, along with normal gamma counts during the resting phase of the test, indicates a partial blockage of one or more coronary arteries. A decrease in gamma counts during both tests indicates more severe blockage of one or more coronary arteries.

Although few studies have been conducted on the accuracy of the thallium exercise stress test in women, existing studies have found the test to be much more accurate than the exercise stress test in detecting coronary blockages. Still, the test is not as accurate in women as it is in men, partly because a woman's breast tissue tends to weaken the gamma counter's ability to detect gamma rays. When this problem is taken into account, however, the test results are as accurate in women as they are in men.

Echocardiogram

This test may be recommended if you have a heart murmur or if your physician suspects that one or more of your heart's chambers or the heart muscle itself has become enlarged (left ventricular hypertrophy). Left ventricular hypertrophy is now recognized as an important risk factor for coronary artery disease. The test uses sound waves from a hand-held ultrasound probe to create an image of the heart's chambers and valves. The echocardiogram is painless, noninvasive, and involves no radiation.

During the test, you lie quietly on an examining table while your physician or a qualified technician places a small amount of gel or mineral oil on your chest. The ultrasound transducer is then placed on your chest in a space between the ribs. The entire test takes about thirty minutes.

CHEST PAIN: MAKING A DIAGNOSIS

Chest pain can have many different underlying causes. Here are examples of three women and how their chest pain was evaluated.

JOAN

Joan came to our clinic at age fifty-four seeking relief from hot flashes and other menopausal symptoms. Joan had no family history of cardiovascular disease, but her total and LDL cholesterol levels were high. She was given combination hormone therapy to treat her menopausal symptoms and to help lower her cholesterol. Joan was also advised to follow a low-fat diet.

Seven months after her initial visit, Joan returned to the clinic complaining of chest pain. She had an electrocardiogram (ECG), which was normal. She then underwent a thallium exercise stress test, which found evidence of coronary artery disease. Since Joan was a possible candidate for angioplasty, she had an angiogram, which showed that her left anterior descending coronary artery was 75 percent blocked. The blockage was successfully treated with angioplasty.

MARY JEAN

Mary Jean came to our clinic at age fifty complaining of an "uncomfortable feeling" in her chest. A physical exam revealed that she had a heart murmur. Other routine screening tests found that she had high triglycerides (426 mg/dl) and low HDL

---

cholesterol (34 mg/dl), elevated blood pressure (146/92), and a positive glucose-tolerance test. Because of her high blood pressure, blood cholesterol, and blood sugar levels, she was given an exercise stress test, which found no evidence of heart disease. She also had an echocardiogram, which found no evidence of mitral valve prolapse or cardiomyopathy. Finally, Mary Jean underwent an evaluation for esophageal pain, which was negative. Mary Jean was diagnosed with microvascular angina, atypical coronary artery pain that may be a result of chest wall spasms or spasms of the coronary arteries themselves.

GLENDA

Fifty-year-old Glenda sought our help for hot flashes and arthritis pain. During her evaluation, she mentioned that she sometimes was awakened at night with chest pain, but didn't think it was anything serious. A physical exam revealed a fairly marked heart murmur, and we recommended that she have an echocardiogram. The echocardiogram revealed severe mitral valve prolapse with significant regurgitation. The left atrium of the heart was also enlarged, but the rest of the heart was normal. Although mitral valve prolapse is not a life-threatening condition, Glenda's was severe enough that she will have to take certain precautions to prevent an infection of the heart valves. (For more on mitral valve prolapse, see Chapter 15.)

Holter Monitor

If you have a heart murmur or your doctor suspects you have arrhythmias or coronary artery disease, you may be asked to wear a Holter monitor. The device consists of a small tape recorder attached to several electrodes that are placed on your chest. The monitor records your heart's rhythm and electrical activity over a twenty-four-hour period while you go about your normal activities.

Cardiac Catheterization

This is the most definitive way to diagnose coronary artery disease. It is also the most invasive test, and the most expensive. For this reason, cardiac catheterization is usually reserved for women who are possible candidates

FIGURE 7 — Cardiac Catheterization

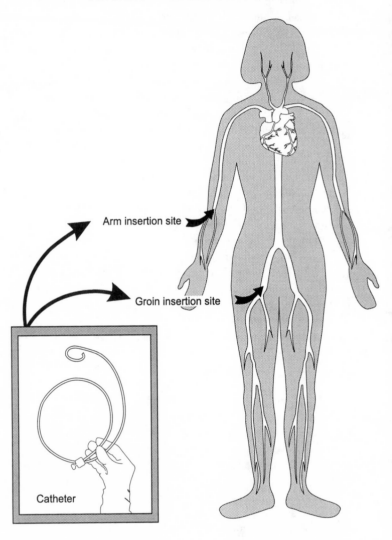

Arm insertion site

Groin insertion site

Catheter

for angioplasty or bypass surgery. Cardiac catheterization is generally conducted only after you have had an echocardiogram, ECG, and exercise stress test. The procedure may be recommended when your doctor suspects you have significant coronary artery disease but other tests don't provide definitive proof, and a definite answer is needed to plan your therapy.

Because it involves many of the risks associated with an operation, catheterization is always done in the hospital under sedation. During the test, one or more catheters (long, flexible tubes) are inserted into an artery or vein (usually in the groin) and guided into the heart (see Figure 7). The catheters may be used to take blood pressure readings, collect blood samples, and inject a dye that makes the heart's chambers and coronary arteries visible on X-ray film. Catheterization is used to help diagnose narrowed or scarred heart valves, defects in the wall between the heart's chambers, the heart's overall ability to pump blood, and coronary artery disease.

Lifestyle Evaluation

As part of a routine cardiovascular evaluation, you should also consider having a nutritional evaluation conducted by a registered dietitian and a formal assessment of your fitness level, which may include an exercise stress test. Your doctor will also want to know whether or not you smoke cigarettes, how much alcohol you consume—and how often—and whether you are under a lot of emotional stress, since all of these lifestyle habits can affect your risk.

Once you have a better idea of your heart's health, you and your physician can concentrate on developing a program of prevention or treatment best suited to your needs.

CHAPTER 6

A Prudent Diet for the Prevention of Coronary Artery Disease

IF YOU HAVE high blood cholesterol, high blood pressure, or other risk factors for heart disease, making healthier food choices is one way you can reduce your risk.

How effective are dietary measures in reducing your risk of heart disease? Most research suggests that you may be able to reduce your total and LDL cholesterol levels by 10 to 15 percent by following a low-fat, low-cholesterol diet. This translates into a 20 to 30 percent reduction in heart disease risk through diet therapy alone—one of the safest ways to prevent heart problems.

Remember, too, that while blood cholesterol levels are the easiest way to measure the relative "success" or "failure" of diet therapy, they tell only part of the story. For instance, some of the dietary recommendations discussed in this chapter protect against heart disease, not by lowering cholesterol, but by other means, such as protecting against the development of blood clots, or by lowering blood levels of homocysteine. So even if you don't see drastic changes in your blood cholesterol levels, your healthy eating habits are likely paying off in other—and perhaps immeasurable—ways. In this chapter, you'll find heart-healthy eating guidelines for women, along with practical tips for incorporating the dietary guidelines into your everyday life.

Are the Dietary Recommendations for Men Suitable for Women Too?

The current dietary recommendations for lowering cholesterol and protecting against heart disease were developed with men in mind. But is what's good for the gander good for the goose too?

There is some controversy about whether women should follow the same dietary recommendations for lowering cholesterol as men. Questions were raised after preliminary studies suggested that the low-fat, low-cholesterol diet now recommended for men doesn't lower blood cholesterol levels as readily in women, or as dramatically. Other studies have suggested that a low-fat, high-carbohydrate diet may actually raise triglycerides. High triglycerides, as you know, are a strong risk factor for postmenopausal women. Another, larger study involving two thousand postmenopausal women found that a very-low-fat diet was associated with a decline in HDL cholesterol levels in women. This was a particularly worrisome finding, since high HDL cholesterol may be more important in conferring protection to women than high LDL cholesterol is in raising a woman's risk.

Before you jump to the conclusion that you don't need to change your eating habits to lower cholesterol, keep in mind that most of the studies so far are small, and can only be considered preliminary. More research needs to be conducted before we have answers to many of these questions. And studies are now underway to determine whether the dietary recommendations for men are equally beneficial to women.

As for the question about triglycerides, researchers point out that high-carbohydrate diets lead to the production of large, buoyant molecules of very-low-density lipoprotein (VLDL) particles, which are believed to be less likely to contribute to the development of atherosclerosis than small, dense VLDL particles. The National Institutes of Health Consensus Development Panel on Triglyceride, High-Density Lipoprotein, and Coronary Heart Disease also points out that "in societies that have a high carbohydrate diet and a low incidence of coronary heart disease, blood triglyceride levels are slightly higher and both LDL cholesterol and HDL cholesterol are lower than in societies that consume a western diet." For these reasons, the standard low-fat, high-carbohydrate, high-fiber diet is recommended for women with high triglycerides, even though the diet initially may increase blood triglyceride levels.

Scientists also point to studies involving both men and women that strongly support the idea that lowering total and LDL cholesterol—

through diet alone or both diet and drug therapy—is just as beneficial to women as it is to men—even though the reductions in total and LDL cholesterol in women may be less dramatic than in men. In several studies conducted in Europe in the late 1960s and early 1970s, for instance, lowering cholesterol was associated with an equivalent reduction in coronary deaths in both men and women. In a more recent study involving men and women with the genetic disorder familial hypercholesterolemia, a combination of diet and drugs was used to lower LDL cholesterol and raise HDL cholesterol. Interestingly, regression of coronary plaques was more dramatic in the women than the men, even though the changes in LDL and HDL cholesterol were the same in both sexes.

Only five women participated in the landmark study by Dr. Dean Ornish, which found that lifestyle changes alone could reverse atherosclerosis. The lone woman in the experimental group, who ate an extremely low-fat diet, exercised regularly, and participated in daily stress-reducing exercises such as mediation, experienced a more rapid and dramatic regression of coronary plaques than the men following the same rigorous regimen. Even more remarkable was the finding that the women in the comparison group, who followed the far less rigorous American Heart Association Step I diet and received counseling about reducing other risk factors, also had regression of coronary plaques throughout the course of the study, whereas the men in the comparison group registered no change in the size of their plaques.

It may be years before scientists have enough information to develop dietary guidelines specifically for preventing coronary artery disease in women. In the meantime, most experts believe there is enough evidence of benefit to women to warrant recommending the current diet low in saturated fat and cholesterol. Besides, there are plenty of other health benefits to low-fat, high-carbohydrate eating. A low-fat, high-fiber diet is the most sensible way to manage your weight, control diabetes, and reduce your risk of several kinds of cancer. So read on to discover how you can reduce your risk.

First Things First:
A Professional Nutritional Evaluation

Change your eating habits and prolong your life. That proposition sounds simple enough. But even with the dietary guidelines in hand, it's not always easy to put them into practice in your daily life. Many people become discouraged when they don't immediately succeed in lowering cholesterol or triglycerides. Women may be especially prone to disappointment if further studies confirm preliminary reports suggesting that their blood lipids don't respond as rapidly or dramatically as men's do.

Many people find it easier to change their eating habits when they work with a registered dietitian or other qualified nutrition counselor. We strongly recommend that you consider this option from the start.

A registered dietitian or licensed nutrition counselor has the experience and equipment to conduct a more thorough evaluation of your dietary needs, and can often perform a computer analysis of your diet. You'll be asked to keep a food diary for five to seven days, logging what you eat and in what amounts. This information is fed into a computer, which calculates the number of calories and nutrients in your diet and produces a graphic printout showing the excesses and deficiencies. Moreover, a dietitian or nutrition counselor also has a wealth of practical tips and suggestions to help ease you into new and more healthful eating habits.

You should be aware that in many states, no special license is required to give nutritional advice, so anyone can call him or herself a nutritionist. Look for a nutrition counselor who holds a Ph.D. or a master's degree in nutrition from an accredited university, or one who is a registered dietitian (R.D.). Ask your physician for a referral, contact a local university nutrition department or community hospital, or look in the Yellow Pages of the phone book. The American Dietetic Association will provide a list of Registered Dietitians in your area. For a referral, call the ADA's consumer nutrition toll-free hotline at (800) 366-1655.

Dietary Guidelines For a Healthy Heart

What constitutes a heart-healthy diet? You may already be familiar with perhaps the most important recommendation: reduce the amount of total fat, saturated fat, and cholesterol in your diet. The question is, *How much fat?* and *How do you make the change in your diet?* Take a closer look at this and other dietary guidelines for a healthy heart, and some of the ways you can start to incorporate the guidelines into your lifestyle.

Fat

Of all the things you can do to lower your risk of heart disease, cutting back on fat in your diet is one of the most important. Population studies show that rates of coronary artery disease are relatively low among cultures that consume low-fat diets. In Japan, where coronary artery disease rarely

FIGURE 8 — Fatty Acids: A Closer Look

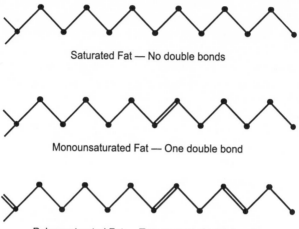

Saturated Fat — No double bonds

Monounsaturated Fat — One double bond

Polyunsaturated Fat — Two or more double bonds

develops, the average diet is just 10 to 20 percent total fat, and average blood cholesterol levels are between 125 and 166 mg/dl. On the other hand, the average American diet is about 38 percent fat, and average blood cholesterol levels are 205 mg/dl.

A diet high in *total fat* is associated with an increased risk of heart disease. But cutting back on the total amount of fat in your diet is just the beginning. As you are probably aware, there are several different types of dietary fat, and not all are equal in terms of their effect on your risk of heart disease. Some are more likely to raise blood cholesterol levels than others, and a few types of fat may actually confer protection. For this reason, you should take a few moments to acquaint yourself with the various types of dietary fat.

Triglycerides. Most of the fats in your diet are *triglycerides,* or chains of carbon, hydrogen, and oxygen molecules. The building blocks of triglycerides are *fatty acids,* each with a slightly different chemical makeup (see Figure 8).

Saturated fats. *Saturated* fatty acids, found mostly in meat and dairy products, are so-called because they are "saturated" with hydrogen atoms and contain no double bonds of carbon atoms. The important thing for you to know is that *saturated fats can raise your blood cholesterol more than anything else you eat.*

Polyunsaturated fats. *Polyunsaturated* fatty acids, found in fish, as well as in corn, soybean, and safflower oils, have several double bonds. These fats have been found to lower levels of LDL cholesterol, which is good. But polyunsaturated fats may inadvertently lower HDL cholesterol too. Still, when you substitute polyunsaturated fats for saturated fats, your total blood cholesterol level usually drops, which is why these fats—in moderate amounts—are considered heart-healthy fats.

Monounsaturated fats. *Monounsaturated* fatty acids, found in olive and peanut oils (and some meats), have only one double bond. Several studies now show that monounsaturated fats are as effective as polyunsaturated fats in lowering LDL cholesterol. Unlike polyunsaturated fats, however, monounsaturated fats have no effect on HDL cholesterol. Moreover, a recent study of nearly five thousand Italian men and women showed that those whose diets were high in monounsaturated oils had lower blood cholesterol and blood sugar levels and lower blood pressure than those whose diets were high in saturated fats, such as butter.

Monounsaturated fatty acids may help protect in another way: They're much more resistant to damage from oxygen free radicals, possibly providing some protection against oxidation of LDL cholesterol. Obviously monounsaturated fats are good for your heart.

Omega-3 fatty acids. *Omega-3 fatty acids* are actually a type of polyunsaturated fat found mostly in deep-sea fish, such as salmon and tuna, and, of course, in fish oil supplements. Omega-3 fatty acids are thought to protect against heart disease in several ways, but probably *not* in the way you think. Many people are under the impression that fish oils lower blood cholesterol. In fact, fish oils may even *raise* your cholesterol levels. Omega-3 fatty acids in fish are believed to protect by interfering with the normal metabolism of blood platelets, making them less likely to stick together and create blood clots. Fish oils may also alter the function of the white blood cells known as monocytes, so that they're not as likely to take up residence in the artery wall and develop into dangerous foam cells. Some studies have also reported that omega-3 fatty acids lower triglycerides.

Trans fatty acids. *Trans fatty acids* are formed when unsaturated fats are hydrogenized, or hardened—as when polyunsaturated oils are hardened to make margarine. Although margarines and spreads are relatively low in saturated fat, the trans fatty acids they contain have been found to raise LDL cholesterol. Some studies have suggested that these fats also lower HDL cholesterol somewhat. Then in 1993, Walter C. Willett, M.D., and other researchers with the Nurses' Health Study, reported that a higher intake of trans fatty acids was associated with a greater risk of coronary heart disease among some of the more than 85,000 women participating in the study.

These findings have cast a cloud over what manufacturers once touted as heart-healthy margarines and spreads, and what consumers began substituting for butter. In spite of these findings, margarine still may be a somewhat better choice than butter. According to research by Consumer's Union, publishers of *Consumer Reports* magazine, margarines and spreads have up to two grams of saturated fat and up to two grams of trans fatty acids per tablespoon, for a total of four grams of "bad" fat, whereas a tablespoon of butter has a whopping seven grams of saturated fat (see Table 5). As a rule, spreads have less saturated fat and trans fatty acids than margarines, making them an even better choice.

Cholesterol. What about *cholesterol*? Cholesterol isn't a fat per se, but a fatty substance found in meats and dairy products, such as eggs, milk, and butter. Remember that cholesterol is found in every cell in your body, and most of the cholesterol circulating in your bloodstream is manufactured by the liver. But the cholesterol in foods affects your blood cholesterol levels, too. Like saturated fat, cholesterol in the foods you eat can raise your blood cholesterol level.

How to Cut Back on Fat

Does all this mean that you'll be protected from heart disease simply by substituting "good" fats, such as vegetable, olive, and peanut oils, for "bad" fats, such as butter and margarine? Not quite. Remember: You still need to reduce the total amount of fat in your diet, since a diet high in total fat is associated with increased risk.

We're not saying you can *never* again eat a piece of bread with a pat of butter on it. But the less fat you have in your diet, the better off you will be. How low should you go? Most health experts agree that the

TABLE 5 — Saturated Fat, Polyunsaturated Fat and Trans Fat Content of Fats and Oils

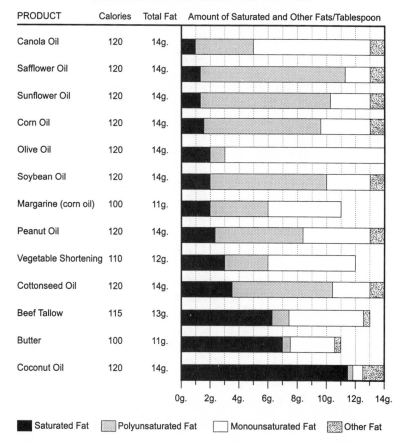

PRODUCT	Calories	Total Fat	Amount of Saturated and Other Fats/Tablespoon
Canola Oil	120	14g.	
Safflower Oil	120	14g.	
Sunflower Oil	120	14g.	
Corn Oil	120	14g.	
Olive Oil	120	14g.	
Soybean Oil	120	14g.	
Margarine (corn oil)	100	11g.	
Peanut Oil	120	14g.	
Vegetable Shortening	110	12g.	
Cottonseed Oil	120	14g.	
Beef Tallow	115	13g.	
Butter	100	11g.	
Coconut Oil	120	14g.	

0g. 2g. 4g. 6g. 8g. 10g. 12g. 14g.

■ Saturated Fat   ▦ Polyunsaturated Fat   ▢ Monounsaturated Fat   ▨ Other Fat

These fats and oils are listed in order of saturated-fat content per one-tablespoon serving.

average American diet, which derives 38 percent of its total calories from fat, is definitely too much. Most major health organizations urge you to reduce the fat in your diet to less than 30 percent of total calories. Of your total fat calories, the guidelines state that no more than one-third should come from saturated fats. The remaining two-thirds should be about equally divided between monounsaturated and polyunsaturated fats. You should limit cholesterol to no more than 300 milligrams a day, according to these guidelines.

Reducing your fat intake to less than 30 percent of total calories is a noble goal—and certainly a realistic one that most Americans can easily achieve. But doing so won't necessarily guarantee that you won't develop heart problems. In fact, most of the studies demonstrating a regression of coronary lesions involved diets containing drastically lower amounts of fat—on the order of 10 percent of total calories. Dietary cholesterol in these studies was limited to 5 milligrams per day. On the other hand, coronary lesions in women appear to regress more readily and with less drastic dietary changes than those in men.

Unless you already have coronary artery disease, we recommend that you start by reducing your dietary fat consumption to less than 25 percent of total calories. If your blood cholesterol levels don't respond in kind, you may want to consider reducing the fat in your diet even further.

You should also work with a registered dietitian or your physician to adapt the guidelines to your particular lipid profile. If, for instance, you have low HDL cholesterol, you may want to have it monitored to ensure that increasing your intake of polyunsaturated fats doesn't lower it even more. Another alternative is to substitute mainly monounsaturated fats and oils for saturated fats, and use polyunsaturated fats sparingly. If you have high blood triglyceride levels or have had a previous thrombosis, you may want to consider increasing your intake of fish to more than twice a week.

If the guidelines sound complicated, relax. There are ways to incorporate them into your diet without too much fuss.

Counting Fat Grams

One way to reduce the amount of fat in your diet is to calculate the amount of fat, in grams, that you can eat based on your total daily calories. All you have to do is keep track of the fat you eat in the same way you count calories on a diet. To do this, you will first need to know how many calories you *should be* eating every day to maintain (or lose) weight. Your doctor or a registered dietitian can help you with this.

Once you know your total daily calories, check the Fat Intake Guidelines below for the maximum amount of fat (in grams) you are permitted each day. Then check food labels or purchase a book that lists the fat gram content of foods to determine the number of fat grams in the foods you eat. When calculating your fat intake, don't forget to count the oil you use in cooking, the mayonnaise you spread on your sandwich, and the salad dressing you use on your fresh greens. And remember not to exceed your total daily calories—even if you don't use up all of your fat grams for the day.

Fat Intake Guidelines

Use this table to determine the number of fat grams you are allowed each day on a diet in which 25 percent of your total calories come from fat.

If your total calories are approximately	Your total fat calories should be	Which converts to (grams of fat)
1,000	250	28
1,200	300	33
1,400	350	39
1,500	375	42
1,600	400	44
1,800	450	50
2,000	500	55

Counting Fat Calories

If you're a label reader, you can calculate the percentage of calories in a product that comes from fat. To do this, you'll need to know the total number of calories and grams of fat in serving size. The percentage of calories from fat equals:

$$\frac{\text{grams of fat per serving} \times 9}{\text{total calories per serving}} \times 100$$

For instance, a two-ounce serving of chunk white tuna (water-packed) contains 2 grams of fat and 70 calories. So the percentage of fat calories is 2 (grams of fat) × 9 (calories per gram of fat) = 18 (fat calories) divided by 70 (total calories) = .25 × 100 = 25 percent of calories from fat. Thus 25 percent of the calories in a two-ounce serving of chunk white tuna are from fat.

Although the U.S. Food and Drug Administration (FDA) recently passed new labeling guidelines to make it easier to determine how many of the calories in packaged and processed foods come from fat, the labels aren't perfect. The new food labels now tell you the number of calories in the food that come from fat (not the percentage), and what percentage of a person's "total daily value" of fat is found in a single serving. The problem is that this figure pertains only to people on a 2,000-calorie-a-day diet. Many women must eat fewer than 2,000 calories per day to lose or maintain their weight, so their total daily values may be lower. In other words, it still may be prudent to do your own calculations.

As a general rule, you should look for foods with an *overall average* of 3 grams of fat for every 100 calories. Of course, some foods will have more than this; others will have less. Your goal is to eat more foods low in fat and fewer foods with a high-fat content, but not necessarily to cut every ounce of fat out of your diet.

Cutting Back on Fat without Counting

By following a few simple guidelines, you'll automatically cut back on fat—without having to count fat grams or calculate fat calories.

Choose lean meats and the leanest cuts of meat. Poultry (with skin removed), fish, and veal are the leanest meats. Also look for lower grades of meat; choose "select" and "choice" grades over "prime" meats, which contain the most fat. Most shoppers usually purchase their meat by cut, not grade, however.

When selecting cuts of meat, keep in mind the following guidelines:

Poultry: Choose light meat over dark. Light meat contains about half the fat of dark meat. Always remove the skin before cooking.

Fish and shellfish: Most fish is low in saturated fat and high in omega-3 fatty acids. While shrimp and squid are relatively high in cholesterol, they're extremely low in fat, so you can still include them in your diet.

Veal: All trimmed cuts of veal (except chopped) are relatively low in fat.

Beef: Round, sirloin, and loin are lowest in fat. Ground beef is high in fat. If you do use ground beef, choose ground round or ground sirloin.

Pork: Tenderloin and leg contain the least amount of fat; bacon and pork sausage the most.

Organ meats: Liver, kidney, brain, tongue, and other organ meats are low in fat but high in cholesterol, so limit your consumption of these meats to about once a month.

Processed and luncheon meats: These are notoriously high in fat *and* sodium. Look for low-fat luncheon meats, such as boiled ham, honey loaf, and turkey breast. Beware of purportedly low-fat turkey and chicken products (bologna and franks). Most contain less fat than all-beef products, but not much less.

Choose low-fat and no-fat milk and dairy products over whole-milk dairy products. An 8-ounce glass of skim milk contains virtually no fat, compared to 8 grams of fat in a glass of whole milk (3.3 percent milk fat).

Limit your consumption of high-cholesterol foods. Eggs, butter and other whole dairy products, red meats, and organ meats (liver, kidney, and brain) are highest in cholesterol. Try cooking with cholesterol-free egg substitutes (EggBeaters, Better 'n Eggs, Second Nature). When baking, substitute two egg whites for one whole egg.

Use monounsaturated and polyunsaturated oils instead of satu-rated fats whenever possible, especially in cooking. Vegetable, olive, and peanut oils should be your first choice, since they're unsaturated fats. Use margarine and spreads sparingly, since the *trans fatty acids* (created when unsaturated fats are hydrogenized, or hardened) may raise blood cholesterol levels. As a rule, soft spreads have less saturated fat and trans fatty acids than margarines (see Table 5 on page 87).

Bake with fruit (or vegetable) puree instead of fat. Carrot cake, applesauce cake, zucchini muffins, banana bread. . . . These are a few of the more familiar examples of baked goods that can be made with fruit or vegetable purees and juices instead of fat. The purees and juices add moisture *and* flavor to baked goods, and can replace part—and sometimes all—of the butter, shortening, or oil in many recipes. Use store-bought applesauce or baby food purees, or puree your own fresh fruit in a blender (ripe or overripe fruit works best). Substitute the applesauce or fruit puree in equal amounts for the oil in store-bought cake, brownie, and muffin mixes.

Eat smaller portions of high-fat foods. This is especially true of meats. You can get all the protein you need each day from just two 2- to 3-ounce portions of meat (plus milk). A 3-ounce portion of meat is about the size of a deck of playing cards.

Use reduced-fat cooking methods. Making a few simple changes in the way you prepare and cook foods (particularly meats) can reduce their fat content by up to one-half. For instance, a fried chicken breast with skin has 12.2 grams of fat. The same chicken breast roasted with the skin removed contains just 4.5 grams of fat.

Trim all visible fat from the meats you buy, and remove the skin from poultry before cooking. Try broiling, roasting, stir-frying, and stewing meats—these are the methods that require the least amount of fat. When possible, cook meat on a rack so that the fat drips down. Avoid pan-frying or deep-frying.

Use fat substitutes sparingly. Fat substitutes may seem like a boon for those who want to cut the fat but not the flavor from their diets. However, many health professionals worry that the fat substitutes may encourage poor eating habits. High-carbohydrate foods, with their complement of protein, vitamins, and fiber, are still a better stand-in for fat-laden foods—even those made with fake fat.

Avoid cream sauces and creamy salad dressings. Use lemon juice and herbs rather than butter to season foods.

Avoid fast-food. Between 40 and 55 percent of the calories in fast-food meals comes from fat. Even such seemingly low-fat fare as chicken nuggets and chicken patty sandwiches often contain ground chicken skin, which increases their fat content. If you do find yourself in a fast-food restaurant, order a salad, low-fat milk, and other low-fat fare, which are finally making their way onto the menus of many fast-food chains.

Consider the no-meat option. Meat is one of the primary sources of fat in the American diet. Many people find that eliminating meat from their diets altogether is the easiest way to cut back on fat and cholesterol. In addition to being low in fat, a vegetarian diet is high in fiber and rich in vitamins, both of which, as you will soon learn, may be beneficial to your heart.

IF YOU CHOOSE A VEGETARIAN DIET

A vegetarian diet *is* good for your heart. In the pioneering study by cardiologist Dean Ornish, M.D., in which lifestyle changes were found to *reverse* atherosclerosis, volunteers ate a strict vegetarian diet, containing less than 10 percent of calories from fat. Moreover, vegetarian diets overall are considered to be healthy—most vegetarians are closer to a healthy body weight, have lower blood pressure, and a lower incidence of heart disease, constipation, diverticular disease, and cancer than non-vegetarians. Still, there are some potential nutritional problems with vegetarianism, most of which can be resolved with careful meal planning.

Although many people worry about getting enough protein from a vegetarian diet, this isn't usually a problem, particularly if you include in your diet low-fat dairy products and eggs. Most Americans consume far more protein than they need. You will, however, have to make sure that you get the full complement of nine essential amino acids your body needs from your diet to function properly. (Amino acids are the building blocks of proteins). Unlike protein from animal products, which supply most or all of the nine amino acids, protein from vegetables is "incomplete," that is, it doesn't contain all of the nine essential amino acids. This means you will have to eat vegetable proteins along with other vegetables and/or whole grains, which is known as *mutual supplementation*. (For instance, peanut butter on whole-grain bread with a glass of skim milk.) If you include milk and dairy products in your diet, getting the full complement of amino acids usually isn't a problem, since these foods supply most or all of the amino acids your body needs.

Another concern will be to avoid nutritional deficiencies, especially in calcium, vitamin B_{12}, and iron. Again, vegetarians who consume milk and dairy products are least likely to develop calcium and vitamin B_{12} deficiencies, since milk and dairy products usually supply adequate amounts of calcium and vitamin B_{12}. Getting enough iron may still be a problem for non-meat-eaters—particularly for women who are menstruating—since the iron in vegetables is not as readily absorbed by the

Another Way to Cut Back on Fat:
The Cholesterol-Saturated Fat Index

Many people confuse cholesterol and saturated fat, thinking they're one
and the same. But they're not. Remember, saturated fat is a type of fatty
acid that's generally solid at room temperature. Cholesterol is a fatty
substance found in all animal products—meats, milk, eggs, cheeses, and
seafood. *Both* saturated fat and cholesterol in foods can raise your blood
cholesterol level. But saturated fat is particularly adept at it.

The problem is that some vegetable fats, such as chocolate, hydrogenated vegetable shortenings, palm oil, and coconut oil, are high in saturated fat but free of cholesterol. Some shellfish, such as shrimp, crab, and
lobster, are high in cholesterol but very low in saturated fat. Confounding
matters even further are products on your supermarket shelf whose labels
boast, "low cholesterol" or "no cholesterol." Many of these same products
are quite high in saturated fat, and can still raise your blood cholesterol
level.

To help resolve this dilemma and help you make wise food choices,
researchers Sonja L. Connor and William E. Connor at the Oregon Health
Sciences University in Portland, developed the Cholesterol-Saturated Fat
Index (CSI). Essentially, they assigned a CSI value to various types of
food—the higher the CSI, the more likely the food is to promote the
development of atherosclerosis (see Table 6). For instance, a 3.5-ounce
portion of cooked fish contains 66 mg of cholesterol and .20 grams of
saturated fat, compared with 96 mg of cholesterol and 8.1 grams of
saturated fat in 3.5 ounces of 20-percent-fat cooked beef. The CSI for the
fish is 4; the CSI for the beef is 13.

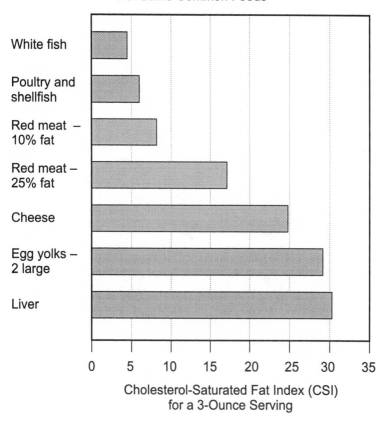

TABLE 6 — The Cholesterol-Saturated Fat Index
of Some Common Foods

Cholesterol-Saturated Fat Index (CSI)
for a 3-Ounce Serving

Shellfish has been much maligned among the cholesterol-conscious because it contains a relatively high amount of cholesterol. Yet it's low in saturated fat. When both cholesterol and saturated fat are taken into consideration, shellfish has a CSI of 6—the same as poultry—and is actually a better choice than even low-fat (10-percent-fat) red meats.

The Connors' Cholesterol-Saturated Fat Index is fully described in their book, *The New American Diet System* (New York: Simon & Schuster Fireside, 1992), which also includes hundreds of recipes and tips for eating out.

Complex Carbohydrates

If meat is taking up less and less space on your plate, what should be taking its place? Complex carbohydrates, such as potatoes, rice, pasta, bulgur, couscous, millet, corn, peas, and beans, as well as fruits and vegetables. These foods are naturally low in fat. Moreover, when consumed mainly in their unrefined state, complex carbohydrates provide protein, dozens of vitamins and minerals, and plenty of dietary fiber, a nutrient that is receiving increasing attention for its possible role in preventing heart disease.

Fiber is the indigestible part of fruits, vegetables, and grains. There are two kinds: *water-insoluble fiber*, found predominantly in whole-wheat products, wheat bran, and fruit and vegetable skins, and *water-soluble fiber*, found in oat bran cereals, oatmeal, dried peas and beans, and barley.

Experts have long recognized the ability of insoluble fiber to help relieve constipation, and to prevent hemorrhoids and diverticuli (painful pouchlike sacs in the colon). Some studies suggest that insoluble fiber may be instrumental in preventing colon cancer too. More recently, the focus has been on water-soluble fiber and its potential for reducing blood cholesterol. Several studies have suggested that when oat bran and other foods high in soluble fiber are added to a low-fat diet, they can lower blood cholesterol levels.

Many of the early studies on oat bran's cholesterol-lowering effect involved men with hypercholesterolemia, an inherited form of dangerously high blood cholesterol. The results of these studies were impressive: in one study, men who augmented their low-fat diets with 100 grams of oat bran per day reduced their total cholesterol by an average of 19 percent. Critics worried about the hefty—and unrealistically high—amounts of oat bran given to the men, and whether oat bran would lower cholesterol equally well in healthy people.

Responding to these criticisms, Northwestern University researchers set out to find some answers. Their study involved 208 healthy men and women and more reasonable amounts of oat bran. The researchers reported a more modest 3 percent decline in total cholesterol when 35 grams of oat bran were added to a low-fat diet. This translates into a 6 percent reduction in the risk of heart disease.

Although one highly publicized study refuted these findings, it's been criticized for its small numbers and poor design. More recent studies support the original findings that oat bran does, indeed, help lower blood cholesterol levels.

The National Cancer Institute and the American Dietetic Association recommend that you eat between 20 to 30 grams of fiber a day from a variety of foods to protect against colon cancer and other illnesses. No recommendations have been made for soluble fiber, since its value in lowering blood cholesterol is still being debated. Nevertheless, complex carbohydrates are excellent, nutrient-packed, low-fat substitutes for the fatty foods in your diet. So by eating more of these foods, you simply can't go wrong.

Simple Ways to Increase Complex Carbohydrates

You can easily eat four or more servings of complex carbohydrates a day from whole-grain foods, fruits, and vegetables, including dried peas and beans. Stick with breads, cereals, rice, pasta, crackers, and other baked goods made from whole grains, which contain the most nutrients. One-half-cup cooked cereal, pasta, rice, or beans; one cup ready-to-eat cereal; or one slice of bread equals one serving. Raw fruits and vegetables contain the most fiber, especially when you eat the skins, peels, pulp, and edible seeds.

Don't feel obligated to load up on special "oat bran" products that promise to lower your blood cholesterol level. More research needs to be conducted before any oat bran products can make such claims. As mentioned earlier, no one knows yet how much oat bran is needed to get a cholesterol-lowering effect. Some studies have found that two to three ounces of oat bran per day (two to three bowls of pure oat bran cereal) is associated with a 3 to 15 percent drop in blood cholesterol. The Northwestern University study found that one bowl of oatmeal, containing just 9 grams of pure oat bran, and one bowl of oat bran cereal, containing 28 grams of pure oat bran, had the same cholesterol-lowering effect.

Remember, too, that oat bran should be used *in addition* to a low-fat diet, not as a substitute for it. In particular, watch out for some of the new oat bran products, including cookies, snack crackers, and chips, which contain enough fat to undo any cholesterol-lowering effects that oat bran may have. Check the label for the fat content of these foods before you buy them.

Keep in mind that several foods besides oat bran are also high in soluble fiber. Barley and dried peas and beans (including black and kidney beans, lentils, split peas, and chick peas) contain the soluble fiber *beta glucan*, also found in oat bran. Rice bran (found in some breakfast cereals) and psyllium seed, the active ingredient in the bulk fiber laxative Metamucil, are also high in soluble fiber (see page 177). *Pectin*, a soluble fiber found primarily in citrus fruits, such as grapefruit, also lowers blood cholesterol. As a general rule, eat a variety of foods rich in both soluble and insoluble fiber (see the box on High-Fiber Foods on pages 99 and 100).

Again, as with most nutrients, more fiber isn't necessarily better. Too much fiber can bind to and hinder the body's absorption of calcium and other vitamins, minerals, and trace elements, so limit yourself to no more than 35 grams per day.

When increasing the fiber in your diet, do so gradually (a gram or two per day) and drink plenty of fluids to help prevent indigestion and gas.

Sodium

You have undoubtedly heard that a high-sodium diet is associated with high blood pressure. In fact, from one-third to one-half of all people with hypertension are salt-sensitive; that is, their blood pressure rises when on a high-sodium diet and falls on a low-sodium one. Many people find that simply cutting back on sodium is enough to keep their blood pressure in check.

According to the recommended dietary allowances, you can get by with a minimum of 500 milligrams of sodium a day (the amount in a pinch of table salt). However, most Americans consume from 3,000 to 6,000 milligrams of sodium a day, not just from the salt shaker, but from hidden sodium in processed snacks, prepackaged foods, and fast foods. A reasonable goal to aim for is no more than 2,500 milligrams of sodium per day.

Here are a few ways to cut back on sodium in your diet:

- Substitute herbs and spices or a salt substitute for salt when cooking.
- Omit salt in recipes and instead sprinkle a little on the food on your plate. Studies show that you'll use considerably less salt this way.
- Use yeast in baking instead of baking powder or soda.
- Avoid processed and fast foods, which are usually high in sodium. If you must buy processed foods, look for low-salt or no-salt versions.
- Avoid smoked, processed, or cured meats and fish, such as ham, bacon, corned beef, hot dogs, pickled herring, and anchovies.
- Buy unsalted potato chips, nuts, and other snack foods. Better yet, have a piece of fruit or raw vegetables instead.

HIGH-FIBER FOODS

	SERVING PORTION	TOTAL FIBER (in grams)	SOLUBLE FIBER (in grams)
CEREALS			
All Bran (Kellogg's)	½ cup	12.9	2.1
Fiber One (General Mills)	½ cup	11.9	0.8
40% Bran Flakes	½ cup	4.3	0.3
Grapenuts (Post)	½ cup	5.6	1.6
Heartwise (Kellogg's)	½ cup	2.8	1.4
Oat bran, cooked (Quaker)	¾ cup	4.0	2.2
Oat bran cereal, cold (Quaker)	¾ cup	2.9	1.5
Oatmeal, uncooked	⅓ cup	2.7	1.4
Raisin bran	¾ cup	5.3	0.9
Shredded Wheat	⅔ cup	3.5	0.5
BREADS			
Bagel, plain	½ bagel	0.7	0.3
Pita bread	½ pocket	0.5	0.2
Pumpernickel bread	1 slice	2.7	1.2
White bread	1 slice	0.6	0.3
Whole-wheat bread	1 slice	1.5	0.3
FRUITS			
Apple, fresh, (with skin)	1 medium	2.8	1.0
Blackberries, fresh	¾ cup	3.7	1.1
Cranberries, fresh	½ cup	1.6	0.5
Figs, dried	1½	2.3	1.1
Grapefruit, fresh	½ medium	1.4	0.9
Peaches, fresh (with skin)	1 medium	2.0	1.0
Pears, fresh (with skin)	1 small	2.9	1.1
Plums, red, fresh	2 medium	2.4	1.1
Prunes, stewed	¼ cup	1.6	0.9
Prunes, dried	3 medium	1.7	1.0
Raisins	2 tbsp.	0.4	0.2
Raspberries, fresh	1 cup	3.3	0.6
Strawberries, fresh	1¼ cups	1.8	0.6
VEGETABLES			
Asparagus, cooked	½ cup	1.8	0.7
Beets, canned, cooked	½ cup	2.2	0.7
Broccoli, cooked	½ cup	2.4	1.2 ·

High-Fiber Foods (Cont.)

Brussels sprouts, cooked	½ cup	3.8	2.0
Cabbage, fresh	1 cup	1.5	0.6
Carrots, sliced, cooked	½ cup	2.0	1.1
Carrots, fresh	1 medium	2.3	1.1
Cauliflower, cooked	½ cup	1.0	0.4
Corn, whole kernel, cooked	½ cup	1.6	0.2
Kale, cooked	½ cup	2.5	0.7
Okra, frozen, cooked	½ cup	4.1	1.0
Peas, green, frozen, cooked	½ cup	4.3	1.3
Potatoes, white, cooked (with skin)	½ cup	1.5	0.8
Spinach, cooked	½ cup	1.6	0.5
Sweet potato, cooked (flesh only)	⅓ cup	2.7	1.2
Zuchini, cooked	½ cup	1.2	0.5
LEGUMES (dried peas and beans)			
Butter beans, cooked	½ cup	6.9	2.7
Chickpeas, cooked	½ cup	4.3	1.3
Kidney beans, cooked	½ cup	6.9	2.8
Lima beans, cooked	½ cup	4.3	1.1
Lentils, cooked	½ cup	5.2	0.6
Pinto beans, cooked	½ cup	5.9	1.9
Split peas, cooked	½ cup	3.1	1.1

Table excerpted with permission from James W. Anderson, Plant Fiber in Foods. Lexington, KY: HCF Nutrition Research Foundation, Inc., 1990. Copyright © 1990 by James W. Anderson, M.D.

Antioxidants

If damage from oxygen free radicals can increase your risk of atherosclerosis, can antioxidants help protect against heart disease? The jury's still out on this question, but so far, there is more evidence to suggest that antioxidants *are* protective than there are studies demonstrating no effect at all. Researchers have found, for instance, that when antioxidants such as vitamin E or the food preservative BHT (butylated hydroxytoluene) are added to LDL cholesterol cells in a laboratory dish, they are completely prevented from becoming oxidized.

Several animal studies—most involving rabbits afflicted with a genetic predisposition to high levels of LDL cholesterol—are even more encouraging. Scientists treating the rabbits with the cholesterol-lowering drug *probucol*, which also happens to be a powerful antioxidant, found that the rabbits develop atherosclerotic lesions much more slowly than untreated rabbits. (Unfortunately, probucol also lowers protective HDL cholesterol among people who take it.)

What about human studies? One of the first, reported in 1990 by researchers at Harvard University's School of Public Health, was a six-year study of 333 male physicians with heart disease. The Harvard researchers found that men who took a 50-milligram beta-carotene supplement every other day had a 50 percent lower rate of heart attack and stroke. Another study by British researchers found a lower incidence of angina (chest pain) among men whose blood levels of vitamins C, E, and carotene were high. The apparent protective effects of vitamin E remained even after the researchers included cigarette smoking, a major risk factor for heart disease, in their data.

In another, preliminary study involving only eight volunteers, researchers at the University of California at San Diego tested the antioxidant properties of beta-carotene, vitamin E, and vitamin C alone and in various combinations. During each phase of the study, samples of LDL cholesterol were isolated from the volunteers' blood and measurements of its susceptibility to oxidation were performed in the laboratory. The researchers found that vitamin E alone decreased LDL susceptibility to oxidation by 30 to 50 percent. In fact, the effect of vitamin E was most impressive when the beta-carotene was stopped.

Then came a widely publicized study by Finnish scientists in the spring of 1994, which reported that beta-carotene did not protect against heart disease or lung cancer in 29,000 male smokers ages fifty to sixty-nine. The study findings were particularly controversial because the researchers found a slightly increased risk of lung cancer among men who took beta-carotene supplements. Some experts interpreted the study results as the closing chapter on the health-promoting effects of beta-carotene: there weren't any.

But the story is not over yet. On the heels of the Finnish report came news from the Lipid Research Clinics Coronary Primary Prevention Trial and Follow-up Study. In that study, researchers measured total blood carotenoid levels among 1,800 men ages forty to fifty-nine whose high cholesterol levels put them at an increased risk of developing heart disease. Thirteen years later, the scientists found that men with the highest blood carotenoid levels had a much lower risk of developing heart disease than those with lower blood carotenoid levels. The researchers pointed out that beta-carotene accounts for only about 25 percent of the carotenoids in the bloodstream. So it is quite possible that other nutrients in the carotenoid family, and not necessarily beta-carotene, are responsible for protection against heart disease. This could help explain why the Finnish study found no decreased risk of heart disease among men who took beta-carotene supplements.

Then came a report from the Cholesterol Lowering Atherosclerosis Study, involving 156 men aged forty to fifty-nine who had had bypass surgery. In that study, men who had a supplementary vitamin E intake of 100 international units (IU) or more had significantly less coronary artery lesion progression (measured by angiography) than did men with intakes of less than 100 IU per day, bolstering the evidence that antioxidants do help protect against atherosclerosis.

Another group of antioxidants that is receiving increasing attention in the fight against heart disease is dietary flavonoids. These compounds are naturally present in vegetables, fruits, and beverages such as tea and wine. In a Dutch study, men who consumed higher amounts of flavonoids (particularly black tea) had a lower incidence of death from coronary heart disease and a lower incidence of death from coronary heart disease and a lower incidence of heart attacks than men who consumed lower amounts of flavonoids.

None of the studies on antioxidants to date have included women, and more research needs to be conducted before scientists are sure of the exact role of antioxidants in the prevention of heart disease. Still, while it's too early to make any specific recommendations about antioxidants (particularly about taking vitamin supplements; see "What About Supplements?" on page 109), it certainly can't hurt to eat plenty of foods high in vitamin E and C and beta-carotene. These include the following:

Vitamin E: halibut, codfish, ocean perch, soybeans, rice, bran, wheat germ, almonds, peanuts, pecans, sesame seeds, sunflower seeds, walnuts, and most vegetable oils.

Vitamin C: citrus fruits and juices, raw leafy vegetables, tomatoes, strawberries, cantaloupe, cabbage, green peppers, and potatoes.

Beta-carotene: carrots, sweet potatoes, apricots, squash, cantaloupe, broccoli, peaches, and other yellow and orange fruits and vegetables.

Flavonoids: black tea, red wine, onions, apples.

DIETARY ESTROGENS: ANOTHER FORM OF PROTECTION?

There is no word for "hot flash" in the Japanese language. And cross-cultural studies have found that only 9 percent of Asian women complain of menopausal symptoms, compared with 55 percent of American women. Could it be that Asian

---

women are reared to complain less? Or could it be something in the food?

Interestingly, researchers now suspect that dietary differences between Asian and Western women may be partly responsible for the vast differences in the incidence of menopausal symptoms among the two groups. Specifically, Asian women consume a diet high in soy protein, and soybeans contain large amounts of naturally occurring estrogens found in plants, known *as phytoestrogens* (*phyto* is derived from the Greek word for "plant").

Phytoestrogens are weak forms of the hormone estrogen that are structurally similar to estrogens produced by the human body. Some three hundred plants with estrogenlike activity have been identified, including carrots, corn, apples, barley, and oats. The best known phytoestrogens, *isoflavones*, are found in abundance in flaxseed and soybeans.

A diet rich in soy protein raises blood levels of isoflavones, exceeding by manyfold the levels of estrogen naturally produced by the body. But what happens to these dietary estrogens in the body is rather complicated. Apparently, these substances have the ability either to block the actions of estrogens produced by the body, or to boost the effects of the body's own estrogens.

In premenopausal women, a soy protein diet containing isoflavones appears to have an antiestrogen effect. A diet high in isoflavones prolongs the menstrual cycle and lowers blood cholesterol levels. Researchers note that the antiestrogen drug tamoxifen, given to breast cancer patients to protect against a recurrence of estrogen-dependent cancers, has similar effects. They suspect that soy protein may provide an alternative means of preventing hormone-dependent diseases, such as breast cancer. Animal studies lend support to this theory. Soy proteins containing isoflavones have been found to reduce the formation of tumors in animals; the higher the doses, the greater was the effect. Scientists also point out that the incidence of breast cancer in Asian women is much lower than that in American women.

In postmenopausal women, whose estrogen levels decline by up to 70 percent, phytoestrogens have been found to help boost blood estrogen levels, and may reduce menopausal symptoms as a result. No one knows yet what effect dietary estrogens will have on a woman's risk of developing heart disease. But it seems reasonable to expect that dietary estrogens would help protect against heart disease in the same way that postmenopausal estrogens do.

More research is needed before phytoestrogens can be used for medicinal purposes. But it soon may be possible to protect against breast cancer, help control hot flashes and other menopausal symptoms, and possibly even protect against heart disease by eating foods high in phytoestrogens.

Calcium

Calcium doesn't lower cholesterol, but it may help control high blood pressure, which is a major risk factor for heart attacks and strokes. Several population studies have associated a low calcium intake with high blood pressure. Moreover, calcium supplements totaling 1,500 milligrams per day have been shown to lower blood pressure in hypertensive men.

There are plenty of other reasons for women to ensure that they get enough calcium in their diets, one of the most important of which is prevention of the bone-thinning disorder osteoporosis. A high-calcium diet may also help prevent colon cancer.

The recommended dietary allowance for calcium is 800 milligrams per day. However, most experts, including the National Institutes of Health, now recommend that *all* women consume even more calcium than this—1,200 milligrams per day for teenagers and premenopausal women, and 1,400 milligrams per day for postmenopausal women.

Most women *don't* get enough calcium in their diets. Among one hundred postmenopausal women we studied, more than half did not meet the 800-milligram RDA for calcium. Only 12 percent met the desired RDA of 1,400 milligrams of calcium that most experts now recommend for postmenopausal women. According to government studies, the average woman consumes a mere 450 milligrams of calcium a day—just a third of what she needs. This creates a *negative calcium balance* of 40 milligrams per day—in other words, your body excretes more calcium through sweat and urine than you consume through foods.

Are you getting enough calcium in your diet? To find out, fill out the Calcium Questionnaire on page 287 of the Appendix. If you are among the majority of women whose diet is low in calcium, follow the guidelines here for boosting your calcium intake.

How to Increase Your Calcium Intake

It doesn't much matter *where* your calcium comes from; only that you get enough of it every day. Contrary to the belief that calcium from dairy products is better absorbed than calcium in supplements, several studies now show that it's the *amount* of calcium and not the source that determines whether you stay in calcium balance (that is, you take in more calcium than you excrete through sweat and urine). Some types of calcium supplements may even be absorbed *better* than food. The important thing is to *take in enough calcium on a regular basis to create a positive calcium balance.*

Increasing your calcium intake by eating high-calcium foods should be your first priority. Food provides other valuable nutrients not found in supplements. Moreover, high doses of almost *any* supplement can cause nutrient imbalances. (Large doses of calcium supplements may interfere with iron absorption and can slow the bone-remodeling cycle.)

Low-fat dairy products, such as skim milk, low-fat yogurt, and nonfat dry milk, are excellent sources of calcium. A single 8-ounce carton of low-fat yogurt contains 450 milligrams of calcium—more than one-third of a premenopausal woman's requirement. Plus, the lactose in milk appears to help your body better absorb calcium.

Dairy products are by no means the only good source of calcium, however. Green leafy vegetables (except spinach and beet greens, whose calcium is bound up and not very available), shellfish, almonds, brazil nuts, tofu, and small fish (such as sardines with their bones) are high in calcium. Added to these natural sources are many fortified foods, including orange juice (Minute Maid and Tropicana), calcium-fortified breads, and even calcium-fortified milk (Calcimilk).

To boost the calcium content of foods, use shredded or grated cheese as a garnish for vegetables instead of butter. Another trick is to add powdered nonfat dry milk to skim milk, coffee, or tea, and to cream soups and casseroles. Nonfat dry milk can also be added to recipes for bread, cakes, cookies, or muffins.

Some foods hinder calcium absorption or cause your body to excrete it. Watch out for the following calcium-robbers in your diet:

Fiber: Dietary fiber binds calcium and prevents its absorption, so limit your fiber intake to no more than 35 grams per day. If you are using calcium supplements, take them at least one hour before or two hours after eating a high-fiber meal.

Protein: Diets high in protein cause you to excrete calcium in your urine. A 50 percent increase in protein above the recommended amount (about 70 grams per day) is associated with a net calcium loss of 32 milligrams per day. This may help explain the finding that vegetarians have higher bone mass than meat-eaters. If you're healthy, two 2- to 3-ounce servings of lean meat or a meat substitute (such as tofu or dried peas and beans), together with protein from milk, is all you need each day. Most Americans consume far more protein than this.

Phosphorus: We're not sure what effect phosphorus has on calcium absorption. Early reports stating that too much phosphorus inhibits calcium absorption proved not to be true. However, excessive consumption of phosphorus-containing foods (particularly soft drinks) may contribute to a rise in parathyroid hormone, which is known to increase bone breakdown, and in a subtle way may lead to the development of low bone mass. Until we know more, it would be wise to keep your phosphorus intake down. One way to reduce the phosphorus and increase calcium in your diet is to substitute milk for high-phosphorus soft drinks.

Sodium: High-sodium diets cause your body to excrete calcium. Unfortunately, many dairy products contain substantial amounts of sodium, and women advised to cut back on sodium inadvertently also cut back on some of the best sources of calcium in their diets. If you're concerned about sodium in dairy products, choose low-sodium cheeses.

Caffeine: Drinking coffee or other caffeinated beverages makes it harder for you to stay in positive calcium balance; a high caffeine intake causes you to excrete calcium. So limit your consumption of coffee and other caffeinated beverages and foods.

B Vitamins

As you may recall from Chapter 4, a deficiency in folate and vitamins B_6 and B_{12} has been associated with higher levels of the amino acid homocysteine, and high levels of homocysteine have been linked to an increased risk of premature heart disease. Although more research needs to be conducted to confirm these preliminary findings, it certainly wouldn't hurt to make sure you consume adequate amounts of these B vitamins on a daily basis. If you eat a balanced diet on a regular basis, one that includes five servings per day of fruits and vegetables, you are probably consuming enough folate and vitamin B_6 to prevent high homocysteine levels. As for vitamin B_{12}, the best sources are meat, organ meats, eggs, milk and dairy products, and fish. Again, you don't need to eat massive quantities of these foods to prevent a B_{12} deficiency. Two 2- to 3-ounce servings of lean meat or fish, along with two or three glasses of skim milk or other dairy product per day is sufficient. As for vitamin B supplements, the Framingham study found that half of the people with the highest levels of these vitamins got them from foods alone, without taking any supplements.

Iron

It is still too early to tell whether high storage iron levels are a significant risk factor for heart disease. Likewise, until more research is conducted, it is difficult to make dietary recommendations.

Certainly premenopausal women, who are at a much lower risk of developing coronary artery disease and at a much greater risk of developing an iron deficiency than postmenopausal women, should make every effort to eat foods rich in iron. And since iron deficiency can be a problem for elderly women (over age sixty-five) who don't always eat properly, these women should have their physicians periodically check for iron deficiency. If they are found to have low iron stores or iron-deficiency anemia, elderly women should be sure to increase their dietary intake of iron as well, and possibly take an iron supplement.

As for postmenopausal women, whose iron stores are usually fairly high, rather than cutting out iron-rich foods entirely, a better strategy might be to eat foods high in vitamins A, E, and C. These foods have antioxidant properties that help protect against damage from oxygen free radicals.

Foods that supply plenty of iron include all types of meat (choose from the low-fat meats listed on page 91), clams, oysters, most legumes (dried peas and beans), and dried fruits, such as apricots, figs, and prunes.

Nuts

What about nuts, most of which are high in monounsaturated oils and the antioxidant vitamin E? Although in the past, conventional wisdom held that these high-calorie, high-fat foods should be consumed sparingly, a few preliminary studies now suggest that many varieties of nuts may actually be good for your heart. The first association between nut consumption and cardiovascular protection came from an ongoing study involving more than 26,000 Seventh-Day Adventists living in California. This group of people typically doesn't smoke, drinks little if any alcohol, consumes meat products less than once a week or are vegetarians, and has about half the rate of heart disease as the rest of the U.S. population. Although the study began in the 1970s, it wasn't until 1992 that researchers discovered a connection between a high nut consumption and a lower incidence of heart disease within the group. Overall, 24 percent of the Adventists consumed nuts at least five times a week, and 34 percent ate them less than once a week. By comparison, another study found that only about 5 percent of American women eat nuts five or more times a week, and 70 percent eat them less than once per week.

During the six years following the dietary survey, the Adventists who consumed nuts frequently had about half the risk of a heart attack or coronary death as those who rarely ate them.

A few other preliminary studies appear to bolster the results of this one. In one study, for instance, thirteen men and thirteen women enrolled in a cardiac rehabilitation program substituted almonds and almond oil for some of their usual calories over a nine-week period. The rest of the diet consisted of grains, beans, vegetables, fruit, and low-fat dairy products, with limited amounts of meat, fatty fish, high-fat dairy products, and eggs. During that time, while the total fat in their diet rose from 30 percent to 37 percent of total calories, the average cholesterol level of the study participants fell by about 20 mg/dl. LDL cholesterol dropped as well. HDL cholesterol remained unchanged.

Yet another study involved men who consumed up to three servings of walnuts per day. The walnuts took the place of other fats in the men's diets and total dietary fat never exceeded 30 percent. During the phase of the diet that included the most walnuts, the volunteers registered an average 22 mg/dl fall in total cholesterol. Levels of both LDL and HDL cholesterol fell, too, by 18 mg/dl and 2 mg/dl respectively.

Nuts are a nutrient-packed food. In addition to being high in monounsaturated oils and vitamin E, nuts are high in fiber, magnesium, zinc, selenium, copper, phosphorus, riboflavin, niacin, and iron. Still, much more research needs to be conducted before we can recommend that you include unlimited amounts of nuts in your diet. Remember, too, that nuts—containing about 170 calories per ounce—*are* high in calories, and eating too many nuts could contribute to weight problems. Steer clear of coconuts; coconut fat contains over 90 percent saturated fatty acids.

Coffee and Tea

Some studies have suggested that regular caffeinated coffee rais cholesterol levels and may contribute to your risk of heart disease ways. Newer studies now show that regular drip-brewed coffee (most Americans drink) *does not* affect cholesterol levels. (Coffee prepared the Scandinavian way—by boiling either whole or coarsely ground beans in water—may raise your cholesterol levels, however.) According to a Harvard University study—the largest and best-designed to date—even three or four cups a day of typical American coffee are safe for virtually everyone, even people with heart disease.

Decaffeinated coffee may be another story, however. Preliminary data from the Harvard study and from a Stanford University study have found an *increased* risk of heart disease among heavy drinkers of decaffeinated coffee (four or more cups per day). Until we know more, drink decaffeinated coffee in moderation (no more than three cups per day).

What about tea? As mentioned earlier, black tea contains a group of antioxidants known as flavonoids, and preliminary studies have found that men who drank two to five cups of black tea per day had a lower incidence of heart disease than nondrinkers.

In a Norwegian study involving 9,856 men and 10,233 women ages thirty-five to forty-nine, those who drank more than five cups of tea per day had lower blood cholesterol levels and lower blood pressure than those who drank one cup a day or less.

These studies, while preliminary, suggest that drinking tea may actually help protect against heart disease. So heat the kettle and enjoy.

What About Supplements?

Sure, it's a lot easier to pop a vitamin or fish oil pill than it is to prepare a vegetable or fish dish. But most experts agree that increasing your intake of antioxidants, B vitamins, and fish oils through food is the best way to help reduce your risk of heart disease. Foods have nutrients in them that supplements do not, such as fiber. Moreover, as the beta-carotene studies suggest, it is not always clear whether the protective effects attributed to certain nutrients are actually the result of other nutrients in foods.

If you do take supplements, you should be aware that megadoses (more than ten times the recommended dietary allowance), particularly large doses of oil-soluble vitamins, such as vitamin A, can cause toxicity and interfere with your body's use of other vitamins and minerals. Too much vitamin A can stimulate bone loss, too, so don't overdo it. You need only 4,000 international units of vitamin A each day.

Researchers studying the homocysteine-heart disease connection are also reluctant to recommend vitamin B supplements without first conducting studies to see if supplements would be effective in reducing homocysteine levels. Until such time, limit yourself to the amount of B vitamins found in multivitamin supplements.

What about fish oil supplements? Again, it's probably better to eat fish rather than pop fish oil supplements. Many of the studies on the benefits of fish oils are still preliminary. Plus, the supplements have side effects, including loose stools, gas, abdominal distension, and a possible increased need for vitamin E. Supplements containing cod-liver oil also contain high levels of vitamins A and D, which can be toxic at high doses. Until we know more, stick with fish—two to three times per week.

Why When You Eat Is Important

Evidence is mounting that *when* you eat may be as important as *what* you eat, and that the American tradition of eating the main meal in the evening may be contributing to a greater risk of heart problems.

Researchers trying to explain the French paradox—why the French eat as much fat as the Americans but are much less likely to die of heart disease—have found that one important difference between the French and Americans may be the time of day in which the main meal is eaten. According to R. Curtis Ellison, a cardiologist at Boston University, the French eat their big meal earlier in the day than Americans do, and are more active after the midday meal.

During a preliminary investigation of various lifestyle differences between the French and Americans, Ellison compared fifty Parisians with fifty Americans. He found that the French consume 57 percent of their calories before two in the afternoon, compared with Americans, who consume only 38 percent of daily calories by 2:00 P.M. What's more, the French return to work after the midday meal and generally don't eat again for another five and a half hours. The Americans, on the other hand, have a snack about three hours after lunch, followed by their largest meal— dinner—only an hour or so later. After dinner, Americans typically engage in sedentary activity until bedtime.

Ellison says the important difference between the French and Americans may not be so much the timing of the main meal as the fact that the French don't eat again for another five and a half hours and are fairly active during this time. "When you go back to work and are active after eating a meal, your body uses some of the fat to fuel your activities. This decreases the amount of fat and cholesterol circulating in the bloodstream," explains Dr. Ellison. On the other hand, if you consume a large amount of calories in the evening and plop down in front of the TV or go to bed, as most Americans do, the calories may be more likely to be stored as fat.

In addition to lowering levels of fat and cholesterol in the bloodstream, the increased activity of the French after eating probably improves insulin's ability to clear sugar from the bloodstream, helping to lower blood sugar levels. Remember: Elevated blood sugar levels have been associated with an increased risk of heart disease. According to Dr. Ellison, physical activity also may have a positive effect on platelets, the cells in the bloodstream responsible for forming blood clots.

Dr. Ellison says his theory is just that—a theory—and that more research needs to be conducted before it can be proven. But other researchers have come to similar conclusions about the American habit of eating around the clock. According to Robert Superko, M.D., a cardiologist at Stanford University's Lipid Research Clinic and Laboratory in California, after eating a meal, the levels of fat (triglycerides) and cholesterol circulating in the bloodstream gradually rise, reaching a peak four hours later—what we call the "triglyceride bulge" (see Table 7 on page 112). This is about the time most Americans are ready to sit down and eat their next meal. So in effect, triglyceride and cholesterol levels of most Americans remain elevated throughout much of the day. Moreover, says Dr. Superko, eating a fat-laden meal or snack late in the day keeps blood cholesterol levels elevated throughout the wee hours of the night. "A big bowl of ice cream before bedtime may be reaching its potential to form artery-narrowing plaques between 2:00 and 3:00 A.M., when you are asleep," says Dr. Superko. As a result, for many Americans, the formation of artery-clogging plaques has become an "around-the-clock affair."

Still other studies have suggested that when you eat a single large meal during the day, certain enzymes undergo changes that encourage your body to store the calories as fat. These changes don't occur among women who eat several small meals per day. So if you starve yourself all day and splurge with a big dinner at night, you may be programming your body to store fat.

More research needs to be conducted before the midday meal theory can be proven. In fact, Dr. Ellison and other researchers have also found other differences between the French and Americans that could help explain the paradox: for instance, the French drink more red wine than

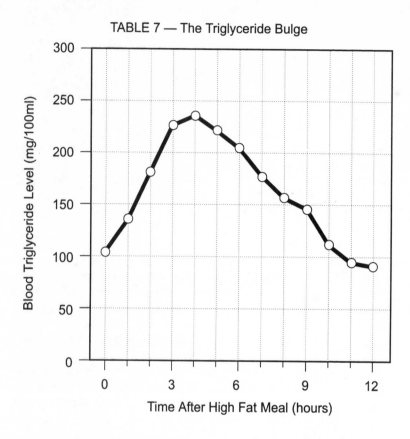

TABLE 7 — The Triglyceride Bulge

Blood Triglyceride Level (mg/100ml)

Time After High Fat Meal (hours)

Americans, and red wine appears to protect against heart disease in a number of ways (see Chapter 8). The French also eat more fresh fruits and vegetables than Americans. As we mentioned earlier, these foods contain dietary fiber, believed to help lower cholesterol levels, and antioxidants, which are thought to help prevent the "bad" LDL cholesterol from forming artery-clogging plaques.

On the other hand, it certainly couldn't hurt to change your eating patterns. We recommend that you eat the majority of your calories *before* 5:00 P.M. This way, the fat in the foods you eat is more likely to be used by your body as energy rather than stored as fat. We call this the PPP Principle: Eat like a potentate for breakfast, a princess for lunch, and a pauper for dinner.

If You Need to Lose Weight . . .

If you are overweight and begin following a low-fat diet and exercising regularly, you may begin to lose weight without even trying. Most people, however, will have to make a concerted effort to get the weight off, and an even bigger effort to keep it off.

It is best to work with your physician and a dietitian any time you plan to lose weight—even if you want to lose just a few pounds. Your doctor can make sure you're in good physical health. A dietitian can counsel you on the most effective ways to lose weight.

If you can't see a dietitian and are wondering how to make sense of the hundreds of diet programs and diet books available to you, keep in mind the following guidelines.

Set sensible goals, beginning with a determination of what you *should* weigh (see pages 64–65). Be sure to discuss what your ideal weight should be with your doctor or nutritionist to ensure that you have set a realistic goal for yourself.

Develop a reasonable time frame within which to lose the weight. A good rule of thumb is to plan to lose between one and two pounds per week.

Don't cut calories too severely. Most adults can safely lose weight on a diet of 1,000 to 1,200 calories a day. (If you have a large body frame or are physically active, you may need 1,500 to 1,800 calories a day.) *Diets providing fewer than 1,000 calories a day can be dangerous and should not be attempted without medical supervision.*

Choose foods high in nutrients and low in calories and fat. Ideal choices are raw vegetables, some fruits, and complex carbohydrates (rice, pasta, whole-grain breads, and cereals).

Take a multivitamin supplement. It's almost impossible to get all the nutrients you need on a diet providing fewer than 1,200 calories a day.

Beware of diet programs promising a weight loss of more than one to two pounds a week. Most of the weight you lose initially will probably be water, which you'll gain right back after the diet is over.

Eat the majority of your calories early in the day. This way, the calories you eat are more likely to be used for energy than stored as fat.

Make regular exercise an integral part of your weight loss program. Dieting alone can cause you to lose vital muscle mass along with fat. Adding exercise preserves—and even builds muscle mass—while helping you to burn fat.

Be prepared to change your eating and exercise habits permanently. See the guidelines below for help.

Changing Your Eating Habits to Last a Lifetime

As you can see, healthy eating plays a major role in protecting against heart disease (and treating existing heart disease). But changing your eating habits may seem overwhelming at times, especially when your goal is to make the changes last a lifetime. Here are a few tips to increase your chances of success.

Set goals for cholesterol levels and weight. Work with your physician and nutrition counselor to make sure your goals are realistic. Be sure to discuss a reasonable timeframe within which to reach your goals.

Take your time. Don't try to be an overnight success by making drastic changes in your eating habits. The only thing you will succeed in doing is making yourself feel deprived. You'll be more likely to stick with your new low-fat eating plan if you gradually phase in new eating habits over time. For instance, if you are in the habit of drinking whole milk, ease your way to skim milk by switching to 2 percent milk for a few weeks, then 1 percent milk, and finally skim milk.

Monitor your progress. Have your physician periodically check your cholesterol levels to measure your progress.

Don't give up! Eating foods high in saturated fat and cholesterol for one day or at one meal won't raise your blood cholesterol levels. But resuming your old eating habits will. If you slip up now and then, don't throw your hands up in despair. Just work your way back into your new eating habits as soon as you can.

A PRUDENT DIET FOR HEART DISEASE PREVENTION

- Reduce the amount of total and saturated fat and cholesterol in your diet. No more than 25 percent of your total
  daily calories should come from fat. Less than 10 percent
  of those calories should come from saturated fats, found
  mostly in meats, milk, and butter. Another 10 percent
  should be comprised of polyunsaturated oils (corn, safflower, and sunflower oils). The rest should be made up
  of monounsaturated oils, such as olive and peanut oils.
  Remember, too, that monounsaturated oils may protect
  against damage from oxygen free radicals, so use these oils
  whenever you possibly can. Limit the amount of cholesterol
  you eat to no more than 300 milligrams per day.
- Eat foods high in soluble fiber (up to 35 grams) every day
  to help keep LDL cholesterol levels in check. These include
  dried peas and beans and, yes, even oat bran.
- Eat foods high in beta-carotene and other antioxidants.
  Yellow and orange fruits and vegetables are chock-full of
  these nutrients, which, like olive oil, may protect against
  damage from oxygen free radicals.
- Drink coffee in moderation (no more than three cups per
  day)—and try to avoid or cut down consumption of *decaffeinated* coffee.
- Limit the amount of sodium in your diet to about 1 teaspoon (2,000 milligrams) per day to help control your
  blood pressure.
- Eat plenty of calcium-rich foods. A high-calcium diet
  (1,500 milligrams per day) may help prevent hypertension.
- Eat fish at least twice a week. Fish and fish oils may help
  protect against blood clots.
- Drink alcohol only in moderation (no more than two drinks
  per day).
- Eat several small meals throughout the day instead of
  three large meals. To help avoid the "triglyceride bulge,"
  consume the majority of your calories before 5:00 P.M. so
  that they're more likely to be used for energy than stored
  as fat, and possibly as cholesterol deposits, in your arteries.

Be patient. It takes time to make dietary changes, and even more time to see the results of those changes. It may be six months to a year before you see a significant change in your blood cholesterol levels. You may find, too, that you have to reduce the fat in your diet to less than 30 percent of total calories in order to see a measurable difference in your cholesterol levels.

Most women who follow the guidelines outlined here will eventually experience a drop in their blood cholesterol levels and their risk of heart disease. You can, too!

CHAPTER 7

Exercising Your Option for a Healthier Heart

CHOLESTEROL GETS all the attention these days, but a growing number of studies now show that sedentary living significantly raises your risk of developing coronary heart disease—perhaps as much as high blood pressure, high blood cholesterol, and cigarette smoking, the three major risk factors for heart disease. University of North Carolina researchers have found that sedentary women are three times more likely to die prematurely of heart attacks than physically active women.

Conversely, regular physical activity appears to be a powerful deterrent against heart disease. A major study by Steven Blair and associates at the prestigious Institute for Aerobics Research in Dallas, found that regular physical activity was associated with lower death rates from all causes (including cancer, accidents, and so forth). But the biggest decline was in deaths caused by heart attacks. The researchers concluded that even if you have another risk factor for heart disease—high blood cholesterol, for instance—you could reduce your risk of dying of a heart attack by almost 50 percent simply by becoming physically fit.

How Exercise Protects Your Heart

Exercise protects your heart in several ways:

- A regular program of aerobic exercise lowers your blood pressure and heart rate, allowing the heart to pump blood more efficiently. Numerous studies, including our own, have shown that *exercise can be as effective as drugs as a treatment for mild hypertension.* In one study involving both men and women, ten to twenty weeks of exercise training decreased systolic blood pressure by 15 points and diastolic pressure by 10 points.

- Exercise burns body fat, which helps counter obesity. Excess body fat is a serious risk factor for heart disease. Studies have found that leisure time physical activities are strong predictors of both waist-to-hip ratio and percentage of body fat in women—the greater the amount of leisure-time activity, the lower the waist-to-hip ratio and amount of body fat. In fact, some researchers suggest that physical inactivity is the most common cause of obesity in women.

- Your body uses insulin more efficiently when you exercise. Our research and that of others has shown that exercise improves your body's ability to clear sugars from the bloodstream (glucose tolerance) and increases insulin sensitivity. Most of the studies so far have involved men; we demonstrated that the same was true for women, too. These changes appear to reduce your risk of developing non–insulin-dependent diabetes (and possibly Syndrome X).

- Exercise raises levels of protective HDL cholesterol and lowers LDL cholesterol. The effect of exercise on blood lipids isn't as dramatic in women as it is in men, but many studies have found that women who engage in regular physical activities (especially endurance exercises, such as jogging) have a more favorable lipid profile than inactive women.

- Preliminary evidence suggests that exercise may also help prevent blood clots. Studies in men have demonstrated that regular exercise raises levels of plasminogen, an anticoagulant that may protect against the formation of blood clots.

- Finally, exercise reduces stress, which may contribute to an increased risk of heart disease.

What Kind of Exercise Is Best?

For protection against heart disease, *any* kind of physical activity is better than none. In one study conducted on Harvard University alumni, even leisure-time activities such as gardening and bowling conferred some protection (although the study involved men only). However, some activities are clearly better than others. We recommend aerobic activities—those that involve increasing your heart rate and breathing and that use the large muscles of your body. When you engage in aerobic exercise, your body undergoes a complex series of chemical changes that overall contributes to improved health and fitness. As you exercise, your lungs take in more oxygen and your heart beats faster to speed oxygen-rich blood to your working muscles. After two minutes of exercise, your body begins the complex metabolic process of releasing stored energy in the muscles (glycogen) and fat tissues. Your endocrine (glandular) system responds to these changes by adjusting the levels of several hormones in the blood, including insulin. Your central nervous system comes into play as it coordinates the movement of your muscles during exercise.

When you exercise regularly over a period of time (three months or more), your heart and lungs become more efficient at what they do and your resting heart rate and blood pressure fall, which helps explain why aerobic exercise reduces your risk of heart disease. Your body's tissues become more sensitive to insulin, protecting you against insulin resistance and non–insulin-dependent diabetes. And since aerobic activities build muscle and rely partly on body fat for the energy needed to sustain them, your ratio of lean muscle to fat improves as well. Many aerobic exercises, such as walking, hiking, rowing, jogging or running, bicycling, tennis, and other racquet sports also stimulate the growth of new bone.

Brisk walking, bicycling, and swimming are ideal for beginners and for women in midlife. Jogging, aerobic dance, and cross-country skiing involve a greater risk of injury and are better suited for women who are already physically fit.

What about nonaerobic activities, such as weight lifting? Resistance weight training has usually been considered dangerous for people with hypertension because weight lifting can temporarily raise systolic blood pressure to up to 200 points even in people with normal blood pressure. Now there is some preliminary evidence that, in men at least, resistance weight training may help maintain low blood pressure. In one study, men with borderline hypertension had a modest reduction in diastolic blood pressure following a nine-week circuit weight training program. In another, a small group of adolescent boys with hypertension decreased their systolic pressure by 17 points and their diastolic pressure by 6 points after a short endurance training program. The boys maintained their lower blood pressure for up to twenty weeks after completing the training program. No studies have been conducted on the effects of weight training programs on women with hypertension.

As for weight control, again, few studies have been conducted in women, but preliminary results suggest that weight training doesn't burn enough calories to be an efficient way to lose weight.

What about the effect of weight training on blood lipids? Of the handful of studies completed, results were mixed. One study found that lean women bodybuilders had HDL levels similar to those of a group of lean, aerobically trained women. Another found a decrease in LDL and triglyceride levels among women who participated in a weight-lifting program three times a week for sixteen weeks. Yet another found no changes in blood lipid levels among overweight women who engaged in a weight training program.

So far, it looks as though weight training does little to increase the efficiency of your heart, nor do muscle strengthening exercises appear to strongly influence other risk factors for heart disease, such as blood pressure, weight, or blood lipids. However, weight training does increase your muscle strength, which improves your ability to do aerobics and decreases your risk of injury. For this reason, we feel that muscle strengthening exercises should be an integral part of a well-rounded fitness program.

How Much Exercise Do You Need?

How strenuously you exercise and how often are also part of the formula for a healthy heart. Most experts agree that you should raise your heart rate to a working level—generally between 50 to 85 percent of its maximum capacity—to give your heart and lungs a sufficient workout. For optimal conditioning, you'll need to sustain the activity for at least fifteen to twenty minutes, and exercise at this intensity three times a week. If you simply can't manage a structured exercise program, the American College of Sports Medicine recommends *at the very least* that you accumulate thirty minutes of exercise through numerous five to ten minutes bursts of activity throughout the day—climbing the stairs at the office instead of taking the elevator, or parking your car a few blocks from your office and walking the rest of the way, for example.

Keep in mind that, you must exercise regularly and fairly intensely before you see a significant improvement in blood lipid levels. And unless you're an athlete, you may be more likely to see a decline in LDL cholesterol than a rise in HDL cholesterol. In one study of ours, thirty minutes of aerobic exercise three to four times a week reduced total cholesterol by about 5 percent and LDL cholesterol by an average of 10 percent, but there was no change in HDL cholesterol. And cholesterol levels improved only after *at least three months of moderate activity*. Other research supports our findings.

Before You Begin

A medical examination is a must before you launch an exercise program. Some women may have certain asymptomatic health conditions (hypertension, heart disease, or asthma, for instance) that could be aggravated by a sudden burst of vigorous exercise. Other physical conditions may limit the amount of exercise you can do or may require that you exercise only under a doctor's supervision. If you have *angina* (chest pain), or other heart conditions, such as *cardiomyopathy*, *thrombophlebitis* (blood clots in the legs), uncontrolled diabetes, or musculoskeletal problems that interfere with exercise, you may be advised not to exercise or to limit the kind of exercise you do (see "Exercise Guidelines for Women with Existing Heart Disease," on page 127).

The examination should include a comprehensive medical history (including a personal and family history), measures of blood pressure, blood cholesterol (preferably a lipid profile), blood sugar, and serum ferritin (women with low iron stores will tire more easily while exercising). A review of your current health habits, including cigarette smoking, alcohol consumption, medications, and diet, should be a part of the examination. If you're over age sixty, you should have your bone density tested before beginning an exercise program.

Women who have one or more of the following risk factors for heart disease may need to undergo additional tests (such as a chest X ray or resting ECG) before beginning an exercise program:

- family history of heart disease
- high blood cholesterol
- high blood pressure

If you are over age forty-five, you should also undergo a graded exercise stress test, which involves monitoring your heart rate and its electrical activity with an electrocardiogram (ECG) while you exercise on a treadmill. The "grade" of the treadmill (similar to the slope of a hill) is gradually increased as the test progresses. As you may recall from Chapter 5, this type of exercise stress test (discussed in more detail below) can detect early signs of heart disease (such as narrowing of the arteries) which may not be apparent during a resting ECG. The test can also determine your level of fitness, your exercise endurance, and your maximum heart rate. Like most diagnostic tests, the exercise stress test isn't perfect. There have been reports of high "false positive" results in women, in which the test indicates heart disease where none exists (see page 74). Nevertheless, the exercise stress test is still a valuable diagnostic tool.

If you're under age fifty and are serious about beginning a meaningful exercise program, you should consider having an exercise stress test as well. As you'll see in the next section, the test is an ideal way to help determine your fitness level.

How Fit Are You?

Besides having a medical examination, it's a good idea to undergo a fitness evaluation to determine your current fitness level and to help tailor an exercise program suited to your needs and abilities. Knowing your fitness level now also helps you set realistic goals and gives you a baseline from which to measure your progress.

A typical evaluation includes measures of body composition, flexibility, and muscle strength. But the single most important gauge of your overall fitness level is cardiorespiratory fitness, measured by *maximal oxygen consumption* (VO_2max). Simply put, VO_2max is a barometer of how efficiently your heart and lungs deliver oxygen to your working muscles, and how effectively your muscles use that oxygen. Scientifically speaking, VO_2max is the point at which your body's consumption of oxygen levels off in spite of an increase in physical activity.

Cardiorespiratory fitness and VO_2max are influenced by your age, gender, heredity, and the amount of oxygen-carrying red blood cells (hemoglobin) you have. There are several ways to measure VO_2max.

Graded Exercise Stress Test
One of the most accurate ways of measuring VO_2max is using a version of the graded exercise stress test called the *maximal exercise stress test*. For this test, you'll be hooked up to an electrocardiogram (a machine that measures your heart rate and it's electrical activity) via a number of "leads," or wires attached to your chest. A small clamp will be placed over your nose and you'll breathe through a mouthpiece connected to a *spirometer*, a device that measures the amount of oxygen in the air you breathe out. As you walk on the treadmill, the equipment will monitor your heart rate, blood pressure, breathing, and your heart's electrical activity, automatically increasing your pace as the test progresses.

The length of the test varies, depending on your fitness level. The test will end sooner if you experience chest pains, dizziness, nausea, or exhaustion, or if the ECG indicates abnormalities in your heart rate or rhythm before you reach VO₂max.

Modified GXT

The maximal exercise test is relatively expensive, fairly uncomfortable, and impractical for use in a physician's office. What's more, the test was designed for use by men. We've developed a modified version of the graded exercise test specifically for women that's less complicated, kinder to the person being tested, and simple enough to perform in a doctor's office. Like the maximal GXT, you'll walk on a treadmill that gradually increases your speed and the slope of your walk while an electrocardiogram monitors your heart rate. Your VO₂max can be calculated with an equation using the amount of time you spent on the treadmill. (Your doctor or other interested health care professionals can write to the authors for more information about the modified GXT, including the formula used to determine your VO₂max.)

The modified GXT is recommended for all women over fifty, or younger women who have one or more risk factors for heart disease.

Bicycle Test

Healthy women under age fifty may take an exercise stress test on a stationary bicycle. During the test, you'll ride the bicycle at a certain speed and adjusted tension for about six minutes. Your heart rate will be monitored by an electrocardiogram, or by a health professional, who will take your pulse several times during the test. The test ends when you reach a specific heart rate or workload, when you feel too fatigued to continue, or when you develop symptoms such as chest pains, dizziness, or nausea. The test results are then used in a formula to estimate your VO₂max.

If you undergo one of the above exercise stress tests, have your physician or other health care professional help interpret the results, and write your VO₂max in the Fitness Profile form on page 292. Use this score as a baseline to measure your progress. To see how your fitness level compares with other women your age, check your score with the Fitness Norms for Women (Maximal Oxygen Uptake) on page 292 and indicate your fitness level in the left-hand column of the form on page 292.

Walking Field Test

Several field tests have been developed to estimate your VO₂max while you climb stairs, run, or walk. While these tests typically aren't as accurate as an exercise stress test in determining your cardiovascular fitness, they can give you a general idea of your fitness level *provided you're under age fifty; you don't smoke, have hypertension, or other major risk factors for heart disease; and you've had a medical checkup and have your physician's approval for beginning an exercise program.*

One of the least taxing field tests is the one-mile walk test developed by researchers at the University of Massachusetts at Amherst and the Rockport Walking Institute. To take the test, you'll need a measured track or other *flat* surface on which you can walk for one mile, and a watch with a second hand (or a digital watch that displays seconds). You'll need to know how to take your pulse, too (see pages 125 and 126).

To take the test, simply note the time you start walking and walk as briskly as you comfortably can. When you've walked one mile, record the time (to the nearest second) it took you to cover the distance, and *immediately* check your heart rate. Now find the charts for your age group on pages 293–295 to determine your fitness level.

Determining Your Maximum Heart Rate and Target Zone

To get a good cardiovascular workout, you'll need to raise your heart rate to somewhere between 50 to 85 percent of its maximum capacity. An ideal training zone is between 60 to 80 percent of your maximum heart rate. This is known as your *target heart range*, or target zone. To find your target zone, use the following formula:

Target zone = (220 - your age) × (.60 to .80)

So if you're forty years old, your maximum heart rate would be 180 (220 minus 40), and your target zone would be between 108 (60 percent of 180) and 144 (80 percent of 180) pulse beats per minute. Write your target heart range in the Fitness Profile on page 292. While working out, you should periodically take your pulse (see "Your Resting Heart Rate," opposite page) to determine whether you have reached your target zone.

Note: Our research has shown that the equation for determining your maximum heart rate (220 minus your age) and target heart range is actually quite accurate among premenopausal women. The formula becomes increasingly inaccurate as you grow older, however: The equation underestimates your maximum heart rate by 9.6 percent in your sixties and by up to 16 percent in your seventies. Essentially, this means that many healthy older women may not be exercising to their full potential or reaping all the benefits of exercise on their cardiovascular system. This is another good reason for women over fifty to undergo an exercise stress test.

Your Resting Heart Rate

In addition to the cardiovascular evaluations above, you should measure your resting heart rate. Although your resting heart rate in itself is *not* a good way to predict your level of physical fitness, it can help gauge your progress in an exercise program. Generally, your resting heart rate goes down as you become more physically fit.

You can measure your resting heart rate any time of day, but the most accurate reading is taken first thing in the morning, before you get out of bed. To find your resting heart rate, you'll need to take your pulse: place two fingers along your carotid artery (at the side of your neck) or on the thumb-side of your wrist (see Figure 9). Count your pulse for 6 seconds. Multiply that number by 10 to determine the beats per minute. Now check your resting heart rate with the Fitness Norms for Women on page 292.

Getting Started

If you have been sedentary for more than a year, we recommend that you start with stretching and muscle-strengthening exercises for the first month or two. For some simple stretching routines to increase your flexibility, we recommend the book *Stretching*, by Bob Anderson (Bolinas, California: Shelter Publications, 1980).

Regular use of circuit weight training machines (such as Cybex, Nautilus, and MedX), under the guidance of a trained instructor, is the safest and most effective way to strengthen muscles, especially if you are out of shape, over age fifty, or have never lifted weights before. After you have built up your muscle strength and flexibility, you can add aerobic activities to your routine. Here are a few examples of beginners' programs for cardiovascular conditioning.

A Beginner's Walking Program

If you are in fair to poor physical condition, begin with a 10-minute walk (5 minutes there and 5 minutes back). Move along at a brisk pace. Add 1 minute each week, gradually building up to a 30-minute brisk, nonstop walk (15 minutes there and 15 minutes back).

Your biggest concern will be ensuring that you walk briskly enough

FIGURE 9 — How to Take Your Pulse

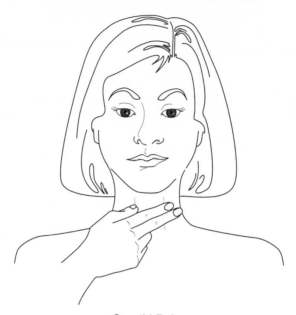

Carotid Pulse

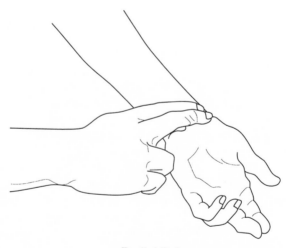

Radial Pulse

to get a cardiovascular workout. Monitor your heart rate while you walk and pick up the pace if your heart rate doesn't reach its working range after 10 minutes or so. For a more intensive workout, swing your arms as you walk, or plan your walk along a hilly route.

A Beginner's Program for Stationary Bicycling

Adjust the bicycle's resistance to the lowest setting. Adjust the seat height so that your knee is slightly bent and just over your toes when the pedal is at its lowest point and your foot is positioned horizontally in the stirrup. Now start pedaling.

During the first week, ride for 10 minutes twice a day (in the morning before you go to work and in the evening when you come home, for example). Then increase the time you spend on the bicycle by 5 minutes each week. When you can ride the bicycle for 30 minutes per session, gradually increase the resistance each week for a more intensive workout. (As you increase the bicycle's resistance, be sure to monitor your heart rate and exercise in your target range.)

EXERCISE GUIDELINES FOR WOMEN WITH EXISTING HEART DISEASE

It may seem odd to you to be advised to exercise when your coronary arteries are impaired in their ability to deliver oxygen to your heart, or after some of your heart tissue has been damaged by a heart attack. But exercise is some of the best medicine for a weakened heart. Regular exercise helps control weight, reduces blood pressure, and may increase HDL cholesterol, reducing your risk of having a heart attack (or of having another heart attack if you've already had one). If you have angina, a program of regular physical activity can actually decrease your symptoms, increase your heart's functional capacity, and enhance your sense of well-being.

Whether you have established coronary artery disease or are recovering from balloon angioplasty, bypass surgery, or a recent heart attack, your doctor will recommend that you participate in a closely supervised cardiac rehabilitation program. These programs include prescribed physical activity tailored to your individual needs. The program may be undertaken in a medi-

---

> **Exercise Guidelines for Women with Existing Heart Disease (Cont.)**
>
> cally supervised setting under the guidance of trained exercise counselors and physicians, in an unsupervised setting, or in a combination of settings.
>
> Before you begin an exercise program, you will be required to have an exercise stress test (if you haven't had one already) to determine your fitness level and your target heart range. (If you already have heart disease, you *should not* rely on the formula on page 123 for predicting your target heart range; it is too inaccurate for people with heart disease.)
>
> The program usually begins with low-intensity exercises, such as brisk walking, two or three times per week. Exercise sessions generally last from 45 to 60 minutes, and include a warm-up and cool-down session. After you have been exercising for a while and have achieved a reasonable fitness level, muscle-strengthening exercises may be added to your program.
>
> You can expect to undergo repeat exercise stress tests six months and a year after beginning your exercise program. These tests can be used to help revise your exercise prescription, assess your risk of future coronary problems, and determine whether any adjustments need to be made in your medication.

Minimizing the Risks of Exercise

One of your greatest concerns, especially if you have an elevated risk of heart disease, is whether strenuous exercise in itself could trigger a heart attack. After all, you reason, doesn't exercise temporarily raise your blood pressure and strain your heart? You may have heard stories of people who had a heart attack while shoveling snow. Does this mean that if you are at risk of developing heart disease or already have heart problems, it would be *dangerous* to exercise?

According to two recent studies, one from the Harvard Medical School, the other from the Free University of Berlin, there is a chance that strenuous activity could trigger a heart attack. But the risk is much smaller than is widely believed. In the Harvard study, of 1,228 men and women who had suffered a heart attack, only 4.4 percent had engaged in heavy physical exertion during the hour before the heart attack. Moreover, those who exercised regularly had an overall lower risk of having a heart attack during heavy physical exertion than those who were sedentary.

The Berlin study confirmed the results of the Harvard researchers. In that study, of 1,194 patients who had a heart attack, 7.1 percent had engaged in heavy physical exertion at the time of the heart attack. In this study, those who exercised less than four times per week had a nearly sevenfold increased risk with heavy exertion, compared with a 30 percent increased risk for those who exercised more often.

Warming up properly before your workout or before any kind of heavy physical exertion, and cooling down after you exercise, can help offset the risk. A five- to ten-minute warm-up of stretching exercises and moderate aerobic activity increases blood flow to the heart and muscles, and reduces the shock of sudden strenuous activity to your heart. Warming up also increases the flexibility of your muscles and joints, which may help reduce your risk of injury.

A five- to ten-minute cool-down period after strenuous exercise is important, too. When you stop exercising suddenly, the extra blood diverted to your muscles during exercise may pool in your legs, causing a dangerous shortage of blood to either the brain or heart. Insufficient blood flow to the heart could trigger dangerous arrhythmias. To avoid this problem, keep moving until your heart rate comes down below your target range.

Much more common risks associated with exercise are injuries to muscles and bones. Although injury may occasionally be traumatic, such as a torn ligament or bone fracture, by far the most common are minor overuse injuries: muscle strains, *tendinitis* (inflammation of the tendons), *synovitis* (inflammation of the synovial lining of the joint, *bursitis* (inflammation of the *bursa*, or fluid-containing membranes in the connective tissues surrounding the joints), and *stress fractures* (hairline fractures of bones).

If you follow the guidelines in this chapter, you will automatically minimize your risk of injury. You may experience sore muscles for the first few days. (Over-the-counter analgesics such as aspirin, acetaminophen, or ibuprofen can ease muscle soreness and stiffness; taking a hot bath before bedtime helps too.) But overall, if you start out slowly, warm up before exercising, cool down afterward, and exercise in moderation, you'll avoid the most common overuse injuries. Don't forget to wear appropriate shoes and use exercise equipment in good working order.

Your body has several ways of warning you that you may be overdoing it. Watch for these signs of trouble during your workouts:

SLOW DOWN: If you experience any of the following symptoms, you may be working out too strenuously. Slow down by training at a lower heart rate and progressing to higher levels of activity more gradually. If symptoms persist even after you've taken these measures, see your doctor.

- Persistent rapid pulse lasting throughout the 5 to 10 minutes of your cool-down
- Nausea or vomiting after exercise
- Extreme breathlessness lasting more than 10 minutes after you stop exercising
- Prolonged fatigue lasting more than 24 hours after a workout

STOP: If you experience any of the following symptoms, *stop your workout immediately and see a physician before resuming your exercise program*:

- Abnormal heart activity, including fluttering, jumping, or palpitations in the chest or throat; sudden burst of rapid heartbeats; or a sudden slowing of a rapid pulse rate
- Pain or pressure in the center of the chest, or in the arm or throat during or immediately after exercise
- Dizziness or lightheadedness, sudden lack of coordination, confusion, cold sweating, glassy stare, pallor, or fainting
- Illness, particularly viral infections. If you exercise when you're ill, you risk developing myocarditis, a viral infection of the heart muscle.

WHAT'S THE BEST TIME OF DAY TO EXERCISE?

You may have heard that heart attacks are more likely to occur in the morning hours. Does this mean it is more dangerous to exercise vigorously first thing in the morning?

It's true that the risk of having a heart attack or stroke is somewhat greater in the morning hours. This has to do with natural variations in the body's chemistry over the course of the day—what are known as *circadian rhythms*. In the morning hours, studies have found, there is an increase in the "stickiness" of platelets, and a decrease in the ability of enzymes to dissolve the coagulant fibrin. Both of these chemical changes increase the likelihood that blood clots will form. Decreased vascular tone and reactivity of the blood vessels themselves during this time of day appears to contribute to the risk.

Maintaining a Fitness Program for Life

To reap the benefits of physical fitness, you have to keep exercising. Months of physical conditioning can be wiped out in a matter of weeks after you stop exercising. For example, 50 percent of the gains you make in an aerobic training program can be lost within four to twelve weeks of inactivity. So you can see why regular exercise and improved physical fitness should be a lifetime goal. Here are a few ways you can help make exercise a regular part of your life.

Set realistic goals. Goal-setting is critical to the success of your exercise program. Successfully achieving a goal you set for yourself can be just the incentive you need to stick with your routine. Write down long-term goals (for instance, how much weight you want to lose), as well as weekly goals—how far you will walk or bicycle during the week.

Start slowly. Beginners often try to get fit in a day, then get discouraged when they develop sore muscles or, worse, suffer an injury. Starting out slowly will keep you from getting too sore or from suffering an injury in the early days of your program.

Choose activities that you enjoy and that are convenient for you. You're much more likely to exercise if you're doing something you find enjoyable. On the other hand, if you love to swim but don't have ready access to a swimming pool, chances are you won't swim as regularly as you should to keep fit.

Vary your routine. Most exercise routines are repetitive, and can quickly become boring. To keep your interest high and minimize burnout, choose more than one exercise and alternate your activity from one exercise session to the next. If your fitness program involves walking, jogging, or bicycling, vary your route from day to day or from week to week to break the monotony.

Exercise with a partner. This way, if your enthusiasm wanes, your partner may provide the incentive you need to go on, and vice versa. Make sure you and your partner are well matched in terms of your fitness levels and abilities, however. It can be discouraging to try and keep up with a runner if you're more suited for a brisk walk around the block.

Monitor your progress. Periodically taking a few simple tests (like some of the self-evaluations described in this chapter) can be motivating, since you'll be able to see your progress. By monitoring your resting pulse rate before you get up in the morning, for instance, you should see a decrease of about one beat per minute every two weeks for the first fifteen to twenty weeks of your exercise program.

Reward yourself. After a month or two of regularly exercising, treat yourself to a movie, a new outfit, or some other reward. Do the same after six months, and again after a year.

Fitting exercise into your life isn't so difficult as it may seem. Just choose activities you enjoy and take it one day at a time. Before long, you'll wonder how you ever got through the day *without* exercising.

CHAPTER 8

Other Ways to Reduce Your Risk

CORONARY HEART DISEASE is the result of many different factors working together, and there are many things you can do to prevent heart disease in addition to eating right and exercising regularly. Here are more ways you can reduce your risk.

If You Smoke

If you smoke cigarettes, quitting may be one of the most important things you can do to reduce your risk of a heart attack or stroke. Numerous studies have consistently found that the risk of coronary heart disease is two to four times higher among women who smoke twenty or more cigarettes a day, compared with nonsmokers. Even light smokers (one to four cigarettes a day) have more than twice the risk of coronary heart disease as nonsmokers.

When you light up, several changes occur in the heart and circulatory system. Carbon monoxide in cigarette smoke reduces the blood's oxygen-carrying ability, so there's less oxygen available to your heart and other organs. Cigarette smoking raises levels of LDL cholesterol and decreases HDL cholesterol. Animal studies suggest that smoking damages the lining of the coronary arteries, setting the stage for the development of coronary lesions. Several human studies have demonstrated that smokers *do* have more, and more severe, coronary artery lesions than nonsmokers.

Cigarette smoking affects blood coagulation in a number of ways: Nicotine inhibits the release of the anticoagulant prostacyclin from blood vessels, which may be one reason blood coagulates more easily in smokers than in nonsmokers. Levels of the blood coagulant fibrinogen are higher among smokers. Platelets in your blood appear to become sticky and cluster. As a result of these changes, clotting time decreases, blood thickness increases, and the likelihood that blood clots will form and cause a heart attack increases.

By speeding up the activity of the sympathetic nervous system, which controls heart rate and other bodily functions, cigarette smoking may trigger coronary spasms, which could lead to a heart attack. Cigarette smoke may also interfere with the electrical activity of the heart, leading to irregular heart rhythms (*arrhythmias*) and increasing the likelihood of sudden death.

What's more, women who smoke experience menopause an average of two to three years earlier than nonsmokers. The earlier menopause puts you at an earlier increased risk of heart disease.

In addition, cigarette smoking may mask the chest pain that is an early warning sign of heart disease. Animal studies have suggested that the nicotine in cigarette smoke affects the nervous system in a way that decreases pain perception. And a preliminary study by North Carolina researchers found that in male smokers subjected to slowly increasing heat applied by a probe touching their arms, the pain threshold (the point at which pain is first felt) and the maximum pain the men could tolerate, were consistently higher after they smoked cigarettes. This may help explain why "silent" heart disease is more prevalent among smokers with narrowed coronary arteries. It's not enough simply to switch to cigarettes that are low in tar and nicotine. Population studies have found that these women are at no less risk than those who smoke regular cigarettes.

The good news is that no matter how long you've smoked, when you quit your risk of heart disease begins to decline. *Within two years of quitting, your chances of having a heart attack will be cut in half. Ten years after quitting, your risk of dying from a heart attack will be almost the same as if you'd never smoked.* Your risk of having a stroke declines as well. So do your heart a big favor and quit.

Quitting isn't easy. In fact, it may be one of the hardest things you do in your life. We now know that nicotine is a powerful, addictive substance—as addictive as cocaine or heroin. However, quitters today will find more support than ever before, from stop-smoking groups to help break the psychological addiction, to nicotine-laced chewing gum and transdermal patches to ease you out of the physical addiction.

Calling It Quits

If you're like most smokers, you probably *want* to quit. The key to success is to develop a quitting plan designed to help you over the biggest hurdles. For women, the biggest obstacles appear to be the following:

The physical addiction. Nicotine, the addictive substance in cigarettes, appears to be much more addictive than previously believed. The Surgeon General has declared nicotine a substance as addictive as heroin. Moreover, women may be more vulnerable to the physical addiction of cigarettes than men. The reason: Men metabolize nicotine faster than women, so it takes fewer cigarettes for a woman to achieve the same blood levels of nicotine as a man. This may be why women purportedly have a harder time kicking the habit than men.

If you are determined to quit, however, you can. Just remember that withdrawal symptoms—cigarette cravings, irritability, difficulty concentrating, sleep disturbances, drowsiness, headache, and stomach upsets—are strongest during the first two or three days after you quit, then gradually subside over the next couple of weeks. *Physical withdrawal symptoms for even the heaviest smokers disappear altogether after a month.*

You'll find it easier to manage withdrawal symptoms as each day goes by. One way to deal with withdrawal symptoms is to occupy yourself with activities that preclude smoking during the first few days after you quit. Go to the movies, take long walks, go for a bike ride. Be sure to get plenty of rest, too.

If you are a heavy smoker (that is, you have your first cigarette within thirty minutes after waking up in the morning, or you smoke more than a pack a day), you may want to ask your doctor about using nicotine chewing gum (Nicorette) or the more recently Food and Drug Administration–approved nicotine skin patch (Nicoderm, Habitrol). Both the gum and twenty-four-hour transdermal patch (which are available only with a doctor's prescription) help ease physical withdrawal symptoms by keeping some nicotine in your bloodstream for several weeks after you quit.

The psychological addiction. When you smoke, you develop not just a physical addiction to cigarettes, but also a psychological addiction. You may use cigarettes to relax or to deal with anger, stress, boredom, or frustration. Indeed, many women report that smoking helps them relieve stress, or handle difficult situations or emotions.

The psychological addiction may be harder to break than the physical one. It may take months before you begin to feel comfortable without a cigarette in your hand. That's why it's important to find substitute behaviors. Here are some suggestions:

- Keep your hands busy. Fiddle with a paper clip, take up knitting, play cards.
- Find something else to put in your mouth: chew sugarless gum, eat carrot or celery sticks.
- Stay busy with activities that preclude smoking. For example, it's hard to enjoy a cigarette while washing the car, riding a bicycle, or taking a shower.
- Brush your teeth often. Enjoy that fresh, clean taste. And go to your dentist for a professional cleaning as soon as you've stopped smoking.
- Spend time in places that don't allow smoking, such as movie theaters, museums, and libraries.
- Ask your friends for support. And, if you must, avoid smokers for a while.
- Limit your alcohol intake. Drinking is often associated with smoking, and alcohol can weaken your resolve.
- Learn relaxation techniques like deep breathing (see page 143) to reduce tension when you feel the urge to light up.
- Avoid eating too much sugar. Maintaining a stable blood sugar level helps prevent fatigue and depression.
- Exercise regularly. This is an ideal way to relieve stress and anxiety.

Worries about weight. Fear of gaining weight is another major stumbling block for women who smoke. But don't let it keep you from quitting. According to the American Cancer Society, only one-third of smokers who quit gain weight. Another one-third actually lose pounds as they substitute exercise for smoking.

As for the argument that gaining weight may be more hazardous to your health than cigarette smoking, by some estimates, you'd have to put on an additional seventy-five pounds to offset the health benefits gained by quitting. On average, ex-smokers who do gain weight put on only about five or six pounds.

There are several possible reasons for the weight gain. Some studies have found that smoking speeds up your metabolism. When you quit, your metabolism may slow down a little, causing you to gain weight in the weeks after you quit. Weight gain may also be more likely if you feel a need to put something in your mouth to replace cigarettes, indulge in extra food as a reward for stopping smoking, enjoy eating more because your sense of taste has improved, or develop a better appetite because your overall health has improved.

Whatever the cause of the weight gain, it can often be easily managed. A few tips:

- Get regular exercise. Exercise burns calories and may help rev up a sluggish metabolism. Walking is especially helpful because it is an aerobic activity that is not too strenuous.
- Drink a lot of water—six to eight glasses per day.
- Substitute low-calorie foods for cigarettes. Munch on raw vegetables, plain crackers, bread sticks, stick cinnamon, unbuttered popcorn, and sugarless hard candies or chewing gum.

Developing a Quitting Plan

When you're ready to quit smoking, develop a clear plan. Start by writing down all the reasons you want to quit. Next, choose a method. By far the most successful way to quit is to go it alone. In one of the largest surveys to date on smokers who quit, more than 90 percent did so on their own, without any help from organized smoking-cessation programs. Smokers who quit "cold turkey" were more likely to succeed than those who gradually decreased their daily consumption of cigarettes, switched to cigarettes lower in tar and nicotine, or used special filters or holders. (If you decide to go it alone, check out the numerous books, pamphlets, videotapes, and other materials available to help you. See Resources and Support beginning on page 256 for a list of organizations that provide free information on how to quit.)

If you are a heavier smoker who hasn't been able to quit on your own, you may benefit from joining a stop-smoking group. These groups meet at least once a week for about ten weeks, providing support and helping you find constructive alternatives to smoking. Local chapters of the American Heart Association, the American Cancer Society, and the American Lung Association offer stop-smoking clinics. You might also check with hospitals in your area.

Heavy smokers may also benefit by using Nicorette gum or the Nicoderm or Habitrol skin patch (available from your doctor), along with individual counseling or group support to help ease the psychological addiction.

Once you've decided on a method, set a quitting date about two weeks away, and circle the date on your calendar. Some smokers find it helpful during this time to switch to a brand of cigarettes that's low in tar and nicotine and to start to taper down. You might also keep a record of when, where, and under what circumstances you light up. This smoker's diary will help familiarize you with your habit and help you find substitutes to smoking after you quit. You should also write down some alternatives to smoking, such as the ones we discussed earlier.

On the day you quit, throw away all cigarettes and matches. Hide all lighters and ashtrays, and follow the suggestions in your quitting plan for coping with any withdrawal symptoms you may experience.

Even if you don't succeed the first time, keep trying. Many smokers attempt to quit at least twice before finally quitting for good. As you learn new strategies for quitting, each attempt will be a little easier than the last and will bring you closer to success.

If You Drink Alcohol

Several population studies have suggested that *moderate* amounts of alcohol (one or two drinks per day) may help prevent heart disease, particularly among women. Alcohol appears to protect against coronary heart disease by raising levels of HDL cholesterol. Alcohol consumption is associated with several changes in blood coagulation, which could also explain its possible protective effect. Alcohol apparently decreases the "stickiness" of blood platelets, and increases the anticoagulant prostacyclin, keeping it dominant over the blood coagulant thromboxane. Alcohol also interacts with aspirin to prolong the time it takes blood to clot. Alcohol lowers the level of fibrinogen, a blood coagulant and potent risk factor for coronary heart disease. Finally, red wine contains antioxidants known as flavonoids, which may help prevent the oxidation of LDL cholesterol, therefore conferring further protection.

Before you raise a glass or two, however, keep in mind that the studies are by no means conclusive. Dr. Meir Stampfer and colleagues at Harvard Medical School found that moderate alcohol consumption among middle-aged women *did* decrease the risk of coronary heart disease and (ischemic) stroke. But in this study, moderate drinkers also had a higher risk of suffering a cerebral hemorrhage, a type of stroke characterized by excessive bleeding in the brain.

Keep in mind, too, that *heavy drinking* (more than three drinks per day) can damage the heart muscle, trigger disturbances in the heart's rhythm, raise your blood pressure, and reduce blood flow from the heart. Heavy drinking also raises blood triglyceride levels.

Until we know more about the possible protective effects of alcohol on heart disease, it's best to limit yourself to no more than two drinks per day. If you currently have more than two drinks a day, try to curb your alcohol consumption. If you find you can't cut back by yourself, this may be a sign that you have a drinking problem, and you should consider seeking professional help.

If You Have High Blood Pressure

If you have hypertension—even mildly elevated blood pressure—it is imperative that you take measures to control it. Remember, hypertension is a major risk factor for coronary heart disease. Hypertension combined with high blood cholesterol is a double whammy: high blood pressure appears to damage the artery walls, which sets the stage for the development of plaques on the arteries.

Fortunately, hypertension is a highly treatable condition, and lowering your blood pressure can reduce your risk of a heart attack by 20 to 25 percent. Your risk of suffering a stroke can be cut by 30 to 40 percent. (For more on the treatment of high blood pressure, see Chapter 13.)

If You Are Overweight

Remember: Even mildly overweight women (those with a body mass index of 25 to 29) are up to forty times more likely to develop coronary heart disease than women of normal weight. (To determine your body-mass index, see page 283 in the Appendix.) Women who tend to put on weight around the waist and abdomen ("apple" shapes) are more likely to have lower levels of HDL cholesterol, and elevated LDL cholesterol, triglycerides, and insulin, and are more likely to develop hypertension and non-insulin-dependent diabetes. The good news is that losing weight is often enough to lower elevated blood cholesterol and blood pressure, and to keep non-insulin-dependent diabetes in check without drugs and their sometimes serious side effects.

Adopting sensible, low-fat eating habits and engaging in regular physical activity are the best strategies for long-term success. In fact, if you have a weight problem, you may find that simply cutting back on fat in your diet and increasing your physical activity may solve it. If these measures aren't enough, follow the additional suggestions for weight management in the nutrition chapter.

If you are more than 30 percent over your ideal weight (or more than twenty-five pounds overweight), and are otherwise in good health, you may be a candidate for a very-low-calorie diet. These diets—which are really modified fasts containing enough protein and nutrients to keep you healthy—provide one of the quickest ways to lose weight. But while the diets used today are much safer than the high-protein diets developed in the mid- to late 1970s, they are not without risks, and they are not for everybody. If you have recently had a heart attack or stroke, suffer from arrhythmias (abnormal heart rhythms), or have had kidney or liver disease, cancer, insulin-dependent diabetes, or serious psychiatric problems, these diets are not recommended. Nor are the diets recommended for women who are mildly overweight.

Even if you are in good health, *you should not attempt to follow a very-low-calorie diet without a doctor's supervision.* A doctor can monitor you for any complications associated with the diet, including dehydration, electrolyte imbalances, orthostatic hypotension (low blood pressure when you stand up), and increased uric-acid concentrations, which could lead to gout. A doctor's supervision is especially important during the phase of the diet in which you return to conventional foods again. Eating too much food after severe calorie restriction can lead to dangerous cardiac arrhythmias.

For the diet to be most effective, your program should include a trained physician, who can monitor your weight loss and ensure that the diet isn't endangering your health; a registered dietitian, who can help educate you about healthful food choices once you begin eating again; and a behavioral psychologist, who can help you change the eating habits that may have helped contribute to your weight problem in the first place.

The long-term effectiveness of these diets is still being debated. Generally speaking, women who exercise regularly and learn new eating habits as they lose weight do better than those who diet alone. However, after the diet is over, many women *do* regain some of the weight they lost.

For severely overweight women who have failed repeatedly to lose weight using very-low-calorie diets and other weight-loss methods, gastric bypass surgery may be an option. But surgery should be considered only as a last resort for people who are one hundred pounds or more overweight and who have a life-threatening complication of obesity that has been proven to benefit from weight loss, such as non-insulin-dependent diabetes, hypertension, or congestive heart failure. If you feel you are a potential candidate for such a procedure, discuss the pros and cons of this type of surgery with your doctor.

If You Have Diabetes

Remember, women with diabetes are just as at risk of developing heart disease as men of the same age. There are several reasons for the increased risk among women with diabetes. High blood cholesterol is more common in women with diabetes, and HDL cholesterol is lower in people with uncontrolled diabetes. Remember, too, that high blood sugar levels may damage the lining of the artery walls, increasing their susceptibility to the formation of plaques. Uncontrolled diabetes may cause blood platelets to stick together more readily, allowing blood to clot more easily.

While diet is a cornerstone of therapy for all women with diabetes, you should not attempt to treat this serious metabolic disorder by yourself. Rather, plan to work closely with your physician (and possibly a registered dietitian), who will develop an eating plan to help control your diabetes. Your physician may recommend that you follow the general guidelines here to help keep your diabetes under control.

Eat several small meals throughout the day instead of three large meals. Nibbling nutritious foods throughout the day instead of gorging on a few large meals helps keep insulin levels at a more even keel.

Eat a diet low in fat and high in complex carbohydrates. Once again, soluble fiber, found in dried peas and beans, oat bran, and oatmeal, has been shown to help stabilize insulin levels among diabetics. (See pages 99–100 for a list of foods high in soluble and insoluble fiber.)

Exercise. Regular physical activity helps your body use insulin more efficiently. We found that women who exercise regularly experienced increased sensitivity to insulin, thus helping to offset the natural age-related increase in insulin resistance that can lead to adult-onset diabetes. More recently, exercise has been shown to help *prevent* the development of diabetes in men. The more active the men were in a fourteen-year study by researchers at the University of California at Berkeley, the less likely they were to develop diabetes. Moreover, the men at highest risk— those who were overweight, those who had had high blood pressure, and those with a family history of diabetes—enjoyed the greatest protection. Among the nearly six thousand men who participated in the study, there was a 6 percent reduction in risk for each 500-calorie-per-week increase in activity level.

Control your weight. Insulin resistance increases with obesity, re-sulting in elevated insulin levels. Losing weight usually increases insulin sensitivity and brings insulin levels down again. Take medication as needed. If dietary therapy doesn't work, your physician may prescribe *oral hypoglycemic agents* to help lower your blood sugar levels. For the 10 to 20 percent of people with non-insulin-dependent diabetes who don't respond to oral medications, and for *all* people with insulin-dependent diabetes, insulin injections are required.

If you don't already have diabetes, but have a family history of the disease, you should have a fasting blood glucose test as part of your cardiovascular evaluation (see page 70).

If You Are "Stressed Out"

Many questions remain unanswered about the role of stress in the development of heart disease in women. But it certainly can't hurt to take stock of the stressors in your life and reduce stress whenever possible. Here are some practical ways to cope with everyday emotional stress.

Exercise regularly. This is one of the most dependable ways to reduce stress. When you exercise, your body produces and releases a group of hormones known as *beta-endorphins*—the same hormones that produce the "high" experienced by long-distance runners. Moreover, the adrenaline that your body gets ready to pour into a "fight-or-flight" response finds an outlet in exercise. When you've finished a workout, your heart rate decreases, your blood pressure goes down, and your breathing slows down.

To alleviate stress, we recommend that you engage in some kind of aerobic exercise (walking, bicycling, swimming, etc.) twice a day: once in the morning and again in the evening (preferably before 8:00 P.M.) for at least thirty minutes per session. Why twice a day? The effects of endorphins, like most drugs, tend to wear off after a while. By exercising twice a day, you get a double dose.

Eat right. It's easy to neglect your nutritional needs when you're feeling stressed, but good nutrition is more important than ever during times of stress. Stress increases your metabolism so your energy needs rise. Eat foods high in complex carbohydrates and fiber, and drink plenty of fluids to avoid the constipation that often accompanies stress.

Practice relaxation techniques. A number of relaxation techniques have been developed to help counter stress. Among them are deep breathing, progressive muscular relaxation, yoga, meditation, and biofeedback.

These techniques can help undo the harmful effects that emotional stress can have on your body. Relaxation techniques have been found to reduce blood pressure by several points when used in the treatment of hypertension—the higher the blood pressure to begin with, the greater the drop that occurs. Preliminary studies even suggest that long-term use of these procedures may *permanently* decrease your body's response to the stress hormone norepinephrine. Try this simple 10-minute relaxation exercise for starters.

A SIMPLE WAY TO RELIEVE STRESS

Sit quietly in a comfortable position with your eyes closed. Briefly tense and relax all of your muscles, beginning with your feet and working up to your neck and facial muscles. Now breathe deeply in and out through your nose. To help clear your mind of extraneous thoughts, repeat the word ''one'' or the chant ''ommmmm'' silently or out loud. Remain in this relaxed state for 10 to 20 minutes. When you are finished, sit quietly with your eyes closed for a few moments. Now open your eyes.

Get plenty of rest. Fatigue can reduce your ability to cope with stress. But if stress is contributing to sleeplessness, your insomnia may become a source of stress in itself. *Don't* rely on over-the-counter or prescription sleep remedies to break the cycle. Instead, try improving your sleep habits by going to bed and getting up at about the same time every day; sleeping in a darkened room with as few distractions as possible; exercising regularly; using your bed for sleep only; and avoiding caffeinated drinks and foods late in the day.

Set priorities. If you feel overwhelmed by the stresses of everyday living (shopping, cooking, caring for children, etc.), try dividing your tasks into three categories—essential, important, and trivial. Don't even bother with the trivial tasks. Delegate what you can of the important tasks, and concentrate your time and energy on getting the essential things done.

Seek out support. Just talking about what you find stressful may help. A steady stream of research over the past several years has shown that social and emotional support can help protect against the ill effects of stress. And while the health benefits of social support have not always been as clear-cut in women as they have in men, again, it certainly can't hurt to reach out to someone in a time of need.

Social support comes in many forms. One way to seek support is simply to open up about your stressors and share your feelings with family, friends, and, when appropriate, coworkers. If you have a problem that you feel is too private to discuss with even your closest friends and family members, you may want to consider seeing a professional counselor. Sometimes, the most sympathetic and helpful listeners are those who share the same problem. In this case, support groups can be enormously helpful. Community hospitals, mental-health clinics, and area churches and synagogues often sponsor support groups for a variety of emotional concerns, such as divorce, single parenthood, or death of a spouse. Or check your newspaper for a listing of local support groups and meeting times.

Set aside some time for yourself—every day. Above all, make time for yourself a priority. Spend a little time each day—even ten minutes or so—doing something you enjoy.

How Not to Deal with Stress

You may be tempted to reach for a quick fix when you're under stress. If you smoke, you take out a cigarette. If you drink, you may increase your alcohol consumption. In the long run, however, these quick fixes only make matters worse. Nicotine, the active and addictive ingredient in cigarettes, promotes the release of epinephrine from the adrenal glands, producing the "fight-or-flight" reaction classically associated with stress. And according to the National Institute on Alcohol Abuse and Alcoholism, you're likely to feel stronger effects from a given amount of alcohol when you are emotionally upset or under stress than you would when drinking the same amount while relaxed. And research has shown that, drink for drink, the hangover you experience during a time of stress is worse than that suffered during normal periods.

When It's More than Stress

Remember, it's still not clear what role—if any—certain personality traits and behaviors have on a woman's risk of developing coronary artery disease. It's even less certain whether or not *changing* those behaviors that have been loosely linked with heart disease in women would actually decrease their risk.

Given the finding that suppressed anger in women has been associated with an increased risk of death from all causes, including heart disease, it may be worthwhile to focus your attention on changing this behavior pattern if it is one that you recognize in yourself. Several self-help books have been written on the subject of women and anger, the most notable of which is *The Dance of Anger*, by Harriet Goldhor Lerner, Ph.D. (New York: HarperCollins, 1989). But you should be aware that changing your behavior patterns isn't always as easy as reading a book, and may even require professional help. At this point, you are probably the best judge of whether the health benefits (both mental and physical) of changing the way you deal with anger are worth the cost of counseling.

Professional help is almost always required for dealing with anxiety and depression, two problems that overwhelmingly affect more women than men. Because these conditions have been associated with an increased risk of chest pain, and possibly heart disease, we urge you to seek the help of your physician and a trained counselor if you suffer from either anxiety or depression.

A hallmark of generalized anxiety disorder is excessive concern or apprehension about two or more of life's circumstances, such as worrying about possible harm to a child, even when the child is in no danger, or being overly concerned about finances for no apparent reason. Physical symptoms include a rapid or pounding heartbeat, difficulty in breathing, shakiness, sweating, dry mouth, tightness in the chest, sweaty palms, and dizziness (the same symptoms associated with a heart attack).

Major depression is characterized by incapacitating feelings of despair and worthlessness, fatigue, lack of interest in activities that usually bring pleasure, inability to get to sleep or early-morning awakenings, agitation, inability to concentrate, diminished interest in sex, social withdrawal, and possibly suicidal thoughts.

Anxiety and depression are not passing moods, nor are they signs of personal weakness, or conditions that can be willed away. Rather, they are serious mental illnesses that can be treated with appropriate drugs, psychotherapy, or a combination of the two. In fact, they are the most treatable of all mental health conditions, so you owe it to yourself to get help.

CHAPTER 9

Should You Take Estrogen?

WHEN ORAL CONTRACEPTIVES were first introduced in the early 1960s, they were heralded as one of the cheapest, most reliable, and reversible forms of contraception available, and their easy availability helped fuel the sexual revolution of the 1960s and 1970s. At about the same time, estrogen was touted as a veritable "fountain of youth" for postmenopausal women, a wonder drug that could keep women looking and feeling "feminine forever."

Then came news that this wonder drug might not be so wonderful after all. First came reports in the early 1970s linking the estrogen in oral contraceptives with an increased risk of blood clots, heart attacks, and strokes among women over age thirty-five. These were followed by studies showing that estrogen, when taken alone by postmenopausal women who hadn't had a hysterectomy, could cause endometrial cancer. Another blow came in the late 1980s, when a well-publicized study found that estrogen might raise a postmenopausal woman's risk of breast cancer.

In spite of its checkered past, estrogen is one of the most widely prescribed drugs today, offering most of the same benefits now as it did back then—freedom from unwanted pregnancy and relief from severe menopausal symptoms. Still, many women today come to our clinic confused, scared, and armed with a healthy dose of skepticism about estrogen. You may be wondering: Does it cause heart attacks? Blood clots? What about the risk of cancer? Should I use estrogen?

Oral Contraceptives

Today's birth control pills are worlds apart from the ones introduced in 1960. Overall, the new pills prevent pregnancy in the same way: When taken on a daily basis, the estrogen and progestogen in combination birth control pills suppress the monthly release of an egg. Oral contraceptives also thicken a woman's cervical mucus, making it difficult for sperm to penetrate. As a final measure of protection, oral contraceptives make the uterine lining unfavorable for implantation of a fertilized egg.

But today's oral contraceptives contain drastically lower doses of hormones. The pills of thirty years ago contained 10 milligrams of progestogen and up to 150 micrograms of estrogen, compared with just 1 milligram of progestogen and 30 to 35 micrograms of estrogen in today's pills. The result is oral contraceptives that are highly effective in preventing pregnancy, with a much improved safety record. In fact, oral contraceptives may well be the best type of reversible contraception for women in their reproductive years—even women over age thirty-five—in terms of both safety and efficacy.

Yet many women are still skeptical about using "the Pill." Most of these fears stem from studies conducted in the 1970s showing an increased risk of heart attack among oral contraceptive users; the older the woman, the greater the risk.

Oral Contraceptives and Cardiovascular Risk

We now know that these early studies failed to take into account the effects of cigarette smoking on a woman's risk of developing heart disease. In fact, when cigarette smokers were removed from those studies, the risk of heart attack in women over age thirty-five was dramatically reduced—in spite of the high levels of estrogen and progestogen in the older pills. Several other studies have now confirmed that cigarette smoking, not birth control pills, is the main culprit.

Still, while the increased cardiovascular risk associated with birth control pills is due *largely* to cigarette smoking, oral contraceptives themselves have been found to aggravate certain risk factors for heart disease. Past studies have associated the progestogen in birth control pills with higher levels of detrimental LDL cholesterol and lower levels of protective HDL cholesterol, decreased glucose tolerance, and elevated insulin levels, all of which raise the risk of heart disease. So questions have remained about the safety of oral contraceptives, particularly in women over age thirty-five, whose heart disease risk naturally increases with age.

Again, most of these studies were conducted with older oral contraceptives containing larger doses of hormones (particularly progestogen) than today's pills. We are among a number of researchers now conducting studies investigating the newer, low-dose oral contraceptives and their impact on various heart disease risk factors. So far, the results are extremely encouraging. Among the findings:

- While triglyceride levels rose and protective HDL levels fell among low-dose oral contraceptive users who were ages thirty-four and older, the altered levels were still within "safe" ranges that *are not associated with an increased risk of heart disease*. Moreover, a month after study participants stopped taking the Pill, triglyceride and HDL levels returned to their pre-pill levels.
- Glucose tolerance fell and insulin levels rose among users of the new, low-dose triphasic oral contraceptives, but again the changes were not serious enough to raise the risk of heart disease.
- As for blood clots, the changes hormones had on blood coagulants were balanced by changes in anticoagulants. So, in effect, the new low-dose oral contraceptives appear to have a minimal effect on the development of blood clots in the veins—usually in the legs (deep-vein thrombosis).

While the risk of developing arterial blood clots (the kind that can precipitate a heart attack or stroke) is very low, these types of blood clots do occasionally occur among women taking oral contraceptives. We don't fully understand how or why these blood clots develop.

One way to counteract this effect is to take a junior aspirin (60 mg) once every three days. Aspirin stimulates the anticoagulant prostacyclin in the blood vessel wall and suppresses the blood coagulant thromboxane produced by the platelets. In this way, aspirin prevents spasms of the arteries and makes platelets less likely to stick together and form a clot.

What about hypertension? Although birth control pills have a reputation for raising blood pressure, the number of women in which this happens is actually quite low: Only 4 to 5 percent of women with normal blood pressure and 9 to 16 percent of women with preexisting hypertension will experience an increase in blood pressure associated with the use of oral contraceptives. Blood pressure usually returns to normal after these women stop taking oral contraceptives.

It's possible that oral contraceptives may even *protect* against heart disease. Animal studies suggest that oral contraceptives, in particular, may have a protective effect *in spite of changes in blood cholesterol levels that would appear to raise the risk of developing heart disease.* In one study, two groups of monkeys were fed a high-fat, high-cholesterol diet—the kind of diet that promotes narrowing of the coronary arteries (*atherosclerosis*) and often leads to a heart attack. One group of monkeys was given oral contraceptives. The other group received a vaginal ring (a small rubber ring inserted into the vagina like a diaphragm) that secretes contraceptive hormones. As expected, the monkeys in both groups experienced a drop in protective high-density lipoprotein cholesterol (HDL cholesterol), which is associated with a greater risk of heart disease. However, when the two-year study was over, the monkeys taking oral contraceptives were found to have fewer and smaller artery-clogging plaques than those who had received the vaginal ring.

In a later study, the researchers expected to find a twofold increase in the extent of atherosclerosis among monkeys taking oral contraceptives who ate a high-fat diet. Instead, they found a *50 to 75 percent decrease in the extent of atherosclerosis—in spite of reduced HDL cholesterol levels caused by the oral contraceptives.* The findings suggest that oral contraceptives—specifically the estrogen in them—protect against atherosclerosis in ways we don't yet fully understand.

Moreover, a large population study has found no increased risk of cardiovascular disease among former users of oral contraceptives—including women who took birth control pills with higher doses of hormones than today's. Dr. Meir Stampfer and colleagues at Harvard University's School of Public Health compared the number of heart attacks and strokes suffered by women who had used oral contraceptives in the past to that of women who had never used birth-control pills. In the eight-year study involving more than 100,000 women, there was little difference in the incidence of heart attack and stroke between users and nonusers.

Birth control pills are now considered so safe that, in 1990, the Food and Drug Administration (FDA) broke the "age barrier" for oral contraceptives by deleting from the package labeling the reference to increased heart attack risks among healthy, nonsmoking women age forty and older.

Over the next several years, new types of progestogen, including *gestodene*, *desogestrel*, and *norgestimate*, will probably make oral contraceptives safer still. Most of the progestogens used today can produce side effects similar to those associated with the male hormone androgen, including acne, weight gain, and negative changes in blood cholesterol levels. However, gestodene, desogestrel, and norgestimate have few androgenlike properties, so these side effects are unlikely to occur.

The Health Benefits of Oral Contraceptives

Of course, one of the greatest advantages of oral contraceptives is their ability to prevent unwanted pregnancy. In theory, birth control pills are 99.5 percent effective in preventing pregnancy. In practice, only about two of every one hundred users will get pregnant each year. Still, when compared to other methods of birth control, oral contraceptives have one of the best track records. You should keep in mind that pregnancy itself carries risks, and, for most women, it is much safer to take oral contraceptives than it is to get pregnant!

When deciding whether to take oral contraceptives, you should also consider the *other* health benefits associated with their use, including the following:

Protection from ovarian cysts and ovarian cancer. Oral contraceptive users are 70 percent less likely to develop benign ovarian cysts as nonusers, and 40 percent less likely to develop ovarian cancer as nonusers. Protection from ovarian cancer begins in as little as three to six months of oral contraceptive use and continues for up to fifteen years after you stop taking the Pill.

Protection against endometrial cancer. Birth control pills provide 50 percent increased protection from endometrial cancer after just one year of use. Effects last for at least fifteen years after you stop using the Pill.

Protection from benign cysts of the breast. Users of oral contraceptives enjoy a 65 to 85 percent decrease in fibroadenoma, a 35 to 50 percent decrease in chronic fibrocystic breast disease, and a 50 percent decrease in breast biopsies, compared to nonusers.

Increased bone mass. Columbia University's Dr. Robert Lindsay found that premenopausal women taking oral contraceptives experienced an increase in vertebral bone mass of about one percent per year. Other researchers have reported increases in bone mass of the wrist among oral contraceptive users.

Protection from iron-deficiency anemia. Women who take birth control pills are 50 percent less likely to develop iron-deficiency anemia than nonusers.

Protection from pelvic inflammatory disease. Oral contraceptive users have a 20 to 50 percent lower risk of pelvic inflammatory disease (PID), a severe or chronic bacterial infection of the reproductive tract, than women using no contraception. This is possibly because of thickening of the cervical mucus, which may block bacterial invasion. Decreased menstrual flow among Pill users may also be protective, since the uterine lining is an excellent medium for bacterial growth. If you do develop PID while taking oral contraceptives, it's often less severe and less likely to cause infertility.

What About Breast Cancer?

Before deciding to take oral contraceptives, you should be aware of the current research and thinking on the issue of breast cancer. Because certain types of breast cancer are fueled by the hormone estrogen and because a woman's age at menarche (start of menstruation), age at first birth, and age at menopause appear to affect a woman's subsequent risk of developing breast cancer, the hormones in birth control pills (and those used for postmenopausal hormone therapy—see page 155) have come under scrutiny. As for birth control pills, the weight of evidence still suggests there's no overall increased risk of breast cancer associated with the use of oral contraceptives. Several major studies involving thousands of women have found no statistically significant link between breast cancer and birth control pills. There doesn't appear to be any increased risk among oral contraceptive users with a family history of breast cancer or existing benign breast disease either. The only group of women who may be at a slightly increased risk of developing breast cancer are young, childless women who take birth control pills for more than eight years. Even so, researchers are quick to point out that the association is weak and study results have been conflicting.

Who Can Take Oral Contraceptives?

Generally speaking, most healthy women, including women over age thirty-five, can take oral contraceptives right up until menopause *as long as they do not smoke.*

If you are over age forty, however, you should be screened by your physician to ensure you don't have any underlying health conditions that may be exacerbated by the use of birth control pills. If you are healthy, the screening should include a lipid profile and a test for fasting blood sugar levels.

If you have a family history of diabetes or have developed gestational diabetes during a past pregnancy, you should undergo a two-hour glucose-tolerance test, in which your blood glucose levels are measured periodically for two hours after ingesting a glucose solution.

If you have previously had thrombophlebitis (blood clots in the legs), you should undergo tests for *prothrombin time* (which helps determine how quickly your blood clots), *fibrinogen* (a blood coagulant), *antithrombin III* (an anticoagulant that helps prevent clots), *protein C* (a natural anticoagulant), and *PAI-1* (a potent blood-clot-dissolving agent).

For added protection against possible increased cardiovascular risks, we recommend that if you are over forty, you take a junior aspirin every three days (under your doctor's supervision, of course), and that you remain physically active, regardless of your age. Regular physical activity is especially important since it has been shown to confer protection against heart disease and since, for reasons that aren't clear yet, oral contraceptives can have a negative impact on a woman's fitness level. In one study of ours, women who started taking oral contraceptives experienced an 8 percent decline in physical fitness over the course of the six-month study.

Who Should Not Take Oral Contraceptives?

If you smoke, you definitely *should not* take oral contraceptives—especially if you are over age thirty-five. Cigarette smoking appears to act synergistically with birth control pills to increase your risk of developing a blood clot, and possibly suffering a heart attack or stroke (see Table 8 on page 154).

You should also consider another form of contraception if you have had breast cancer, a previous heart attack, deep venous thrombosis that *was not* associated with surgery, or liver disease.

Some Commonly Prescribed Oral Contraceptives

There are four basic types of oral contraceptives from which to choose. Each has its advantages and disadvantages.

1. **Monophasic pills** are the easiest to use, since all pills for each cycle contain the same amount of estrogen and progestogen. However, the pills have a higher total hormonal content than other formulations, and higher doses mean a greater potential for side effects and complications. Some brand names include Brevicon, Demulen, Desogen, Genora, Levlen, Loestrin, Lo-Ovral, Modicon, Nelova, Nordette, Norethin, Norinyl, Norlestrin, Ortho-Novum, Ovcon-35, and Ovral.

2. **Biphasic pills** (which are not frequently prescribed) have a lower total hormone content than monophasic pills and more closely mimic the hormonal changes in the menstrual cycle, but they are associated with a greater incidence of breakthrough bleeding (spotting or bleeding between menstrual cycles). Brand names include Nelova 10/11 and Ortho-Novum 10/11.
3. **Triphasic pills** have the lowest total hormone content of all combination oral contraceptives, but these pills contain up to four different doses of hormones per cycle; if you miss a pill or experience other problems, it's more difficult for your doctor to tell where you are in the pill cycle and what precautions you should take to protect yourself from unwanted pregnancy. Brand names include Ortho-Novum 7-7-7, Tridesogen, Tri-Levlen, Tri-Norinyl, and Triphasil.
4. **Progestogen-only pills** ("mini-pills") have the advantage of sparing you from such estrogen-related side effects such as headaches and nausea. But mini-pills are not as effective in preventing pregnancy as combination pills. In addition, your menstrual patterns may be less predictable and you may experience irregular bleeding problems. Brand names include Micronor and Ovrette.

What About Progestogen-only Contraception?

There are several forms of contraception that contain progestogen alone. These include mini-pills, an injectable form of progestogen known as *Depo-Provera*, and a contraceptive implant known as *Norplant*. Overall, these forms of contraception are not as effective in preventing pregnancy as those with a combination of estrogen and progestogen.

As for cardiovascular risks, there are no studies on the long-term risks associated with these forms of contraception. The few existing studies have found that progestogens have no effect on blood clotting. But progestogens have been found to reduce blood flow through the coronary arteries. Whether or not this reduced blood flow is enough to cause cardiovascular problems remains to be seen. And while high doses of progestogen have been found to impair glucose-tolerance slightly, the effect is not enough to increase insulin requirements among women with diabetes.

As for high blood pressure, progestogens alone are the contraceptive choice for women with preexisting hypertension.

The biggest drawback to progestogen-only contraception is that it is associated with a relatively high rate of menstrual irregularities. In fact, this is one of the main reasons women stop using these forms of contraception.

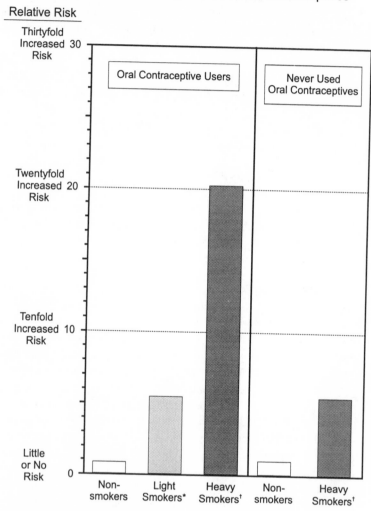

TABLE 8 — Relative Risk of Heart Attacks Among Smoking and Non-smoking Users of Oral Contraceptives

* Less than 15 cigarettes per day.
† 15 cigarettes or more per day.

Postmenopausal Estrogens

These drugs are prescribed to relieve hot flashes and other menopausal symptoms and to prevent the rapid bone loss associated with menopause that can lead to osteoporosis. Now, one of their main purposes is to help prevent heart disease in postmenopausal women.

Postmenopausal Estrogens and Cardiovascular Disease

Perhaps one of the biggest myths about postmenopausal hormone therapy is that it will raise your risk of heart disease or stroke. Mounting evidence now suggests that just the opposite is true: postmenopausal estrogens actually *protect against cardiovascular disease*. In population studies, postmenopausal women who take oral estrogens for ten years or longer have *50 percent less coronary heart disease than women who don't*. And the Postmenopausal Estrogen-Progestin Interventions (PEPI) Trial, the largest and most carefully designed study to date to investigate the effects of estrogen and progestogen on a number of risk factors for heart disease, provides some of the strongest evidence yet that estrogen protects against heart disease. (See "What the PEPI Trial Taught Us" on page 157.) In effect, hormone therapy appears to extend the natural protection from heart disease that women enjoy in their premenopausal years.

Estrogen users appear to be protected against stroke as well: Researchers report a 50 percent reduction in death rates due to stroke in estrogen users compared to nonusers.

How can postmenopausal estrogens protect against heart disease? Remember that most of the research linking oral contraceptives and cardiovascular complications was done on the older birth control pills, which contained much higher doses of estrogen and progestogen than are given to menopausal women. In addition, the estrogen in birth control pills is a synthetic form of the hormone, which has an entirely different chemical makeup from the estrogens typically prescribed for women during the menopausal years. Birth control pills contain higher levels of a different kind of progestogen as well.

Postmenopausal estrogens are thought to protect against heart disease in several different ways.

- Estrogens lower damaging LDL cholesterol by an average of 8 percent and raise protective HDL cholesterol by an average of 15 percent.
- Estrogens don't cause blood pressure to rise, and, in fact, may *lower* it.

- Estrogens don't appear to raise the risk of developing a blood clot. Estrogen lowers the blood coagulant fibrinogen and reduces the stickiness of platelets. These effects are enhanced when estrogen is combined with progestogen. While oral estrogens do raise the levels of several coagulation proteins, these are not biologically active until they're exposed to an injured blood vessel. Plus, "normal" levels for these coagulation proteins vary widely, and it's impossible to use them to predict whether you're at a greater risk of developing a blood clot.

  On the other hand, natural estrogens *don't* decrease antithrombin III, a potent anticoagulant that is a good marker for predicting whether a blood clot will develop.

  In fact, *there is no study showing a cause-and-effect relationship between taking estrogen additive therapy and the development of blood clots.*

- Long-term use of postmenopausal estrogens does not affect your body's ability to use blood sugars (carbohydrate metabolism). Indeed, estrogen *decreases* fasting blood sugar levels, possibly because it prevents the breakdown of insulin. What's more, estrogen does not increase blood insulin levels. Even diabetic women can safely use estrogen.

- Estrogen improves blood flow, and appears somehow to protect the innermost lining of the blood vessel wall from the development of artery-narrowing plaques.

  Estrogen may also protect women against the apparent artery-clogging effects of a type of LDL cholesterol called "small molecule-LDL cholesterol" and against lipoprotein (a).

The Risks Associated with Postmenopausal Estrogens

Over the past several years, headlines that estrogen therapy increased the risk of endometrial cancer and possibly breast cancer spread a wave of fear over women taking estrogens—or those who were thinking about taking them. Let's look at the facts to help dispel some of your greatest fears:

WHAT THE PEPI TRIAL TAUGHT US

Most evidence of a cardioprotective effect by estrogen comes from observational studies involving populations of women who are asked about their health and use of estrogen. While these studies are good at identifying trends and associations, they have some limitations, and generally don't carry as much weight as controlled clinical trials, in which women are randomly given estrogen or a placebo.

The Postmenopausal Estrogen-Progestin Interventions (PEPI) Trial was designed to address a number of questions about the use of estrogen and progestogen in the prevention of heart disease, questions that were beyond the scope of observational studies. For example, most observational studies involved the use of oral estrogen unopposed by progestogen, which is now routinely given to prevent endometrial cancer in postmenopausal women. Would adding progestogen, which is known to affect blood lipids adversely, cancel out estrogen's protective effects? Since past studies associated the use of oral contraceptives with an increased risk of blood clots, what effects would estrogen and progestogen have on blood clotting factors? And since oral estrogens increase the kidney's production of the hormone renin, which plays a role in blood pressure control, would hormone therapy increase blood pressure?

The PEPI study involved a total of 875 healthy postmenopausal women ages forty-five to sixty-four. Over the course of the three-year study, the women received one of five twenty-eight-day treatment regimens: (1) placebo, (2) estrogen only, (3) estrogen plus medroxyprogesterone acetate (Provera) given cyclically for twelve days per month, (4) estrogen plus medroxyprogesterone acetate given continuously for each of the twenty-eight days of the cycle, or (5) estrogen plus micronized progesterone given cyclically for twelve days per month.

Blood levels of LDL and HDL cholesterol were measured at the beginning of the study and several times throughout the course of the study, as were blood levels of the coagulant fibrinogen and blood pressure. Hormone therapy's effect on insulin levels was also monitored.

PEPI taught us several important things about the use of hormone therapy for the prevention of heart disease:

- Estrogen does not lose most of its beneficial effect on cardiovascular risk factors when combined with progesterone. Both estrogen and combination hormone therapy lowered LDL cholesterol by about 20 percent compared with placebo. Moreover, HDL cholesterol was elevated in all women who took estrogen—even in those who took added progestogen—whereas HDL cholesterol fell somewhat (a decrease of 1.2 mg/dl) in women who took a placebo. Among the women receiving hormones, HDL elevations were highest in women taking estrogen alone (an increase of 5.6 mg/dl) and lowest in those taking estrogen along with medroxyprogesterone acetate (increases of 1.2 to 1.6 mg/dl). Women who took estrogen along with micronized progesterone had a 4.1 mg/dl increase in HDL cholesterol.

- Hormone therapy does not raise blood pressure. Blood pressure was unchanged in all groups through the course of the study.

- Women who took hormones had lower levels of the blood coagulant fibrinogen than women who took a placebo. Since increased fibrinogen is an independent risk factor for both heart attacks and strokes, the decreased fibrinogen levels in women taking hormones suggests that hormone therapy protects against heart disease in a variety of ways.

- The problem of overstimulation of the uterine lining by unopposed estrogen, which can lead to endometrial cancer if not treated, is serious enough to warrant the use of an added progestogen in postmenopausal women with an intact uterus, despite the fact that progestogen blunts estrogen's positive effects on HDL cholesterol. Thirty-three percent of the women taking unopposed estrogen in the PEPI study developed this problem.

Overall, estrogen alone or in combination with a progestogen improves blood lipids and lowers fibrinogen levels with little detectable effects on insulin or blood pressure. And this study confirms what observational studies have suggested for some time now: that estrogen and even estrogen-progestogen combinations can significantly protect against heart disease.

As important as this study is, it is still only a start. It is still not known, for example, whether or not the positive effects of hormone therapy on lipids, fibrinogen, and other risk factors will translate into a lower incidence of heart disease among postmenopausal women who use hormones.

It is also not clear what effect hormone therapy has on triglycerides, another important risk factor for heart disease. Oral estrogens have been found to increase triglycerides, and the women taking hormones in the PEPI trial were no exception. Contrary to other smaller studies, blood triglyceride levels rose even among women taking an added progestogen.

Estrogen raises blood triglyceride levels by increasing the liver's production of these blood fats, not by impairing their clearance from the bloodstream. There's some speculation that triglyceride levels elevated by estrogen may not be as dangerous as high blood triglycerides from other causes (such as a high-fat diet). But more research is needed to answer this question.

Another question that we don't yet have the answer to is, how long do women need to take hormones to prevent heart disease? One year? Three years? The rest of their lives?

It will be years before we have the answers to these and other questions about hormone therapy. But the PEPI Trial is a step in the right direction.

Endometrial cancer. The use of estrogen over a long period of time can overstimulate the endometrium. If left untreated, this can lead to cancer. So it's true that estrogen alone can increase the risk of endometrial cancer by about ten- to twenty-fold among postmenopausal women who still have an intact uterus. (During the recent estrogen and endometrial cancer scare, many women who had had a hysterectomy and didn't need to worry, stopped treatment.) However, the absolute numbers are still relatively low: from one case of endometrial cancer per one thousand to twenty cases per one thousand. Moreover, the type of cancer involved is rarely life threatening. It is usually detected at a much earlier stage than some other types of endometrial cancer, and the cure rate is almost 100 percent.

Since the first reports of an increased risk of endometrial cancer associated with the use of unopposed estrogens came out, physicians have begun prescribing progestogen along with estrogens for at least ten days per cycle. This regimen more closely resembles a woman's natural menstrual cycle and prevents overstimulation of the uterine lining by estrogen alone. As a result, the incidence of endometrial cancer among women taking combination hormone therapy *is less than that of women who take no hormones whatsoever.*

Breast cancer. The risk of breast cancer is a concern mainly because of the prevalence of this illness: Now one in nine women will develop breast cancer in her lifetime. The fear of breast cancer was fueled by a 1989 Swedish study involving 23,244 women age thirty-five years and over. While the study showed that women using a combination of estrogen and progestogen experienced overall about 10 percent more breast cancers than expected, the researchers also reported that among the 850 women in the study who took estrogen for nine years or more, the risk increased to 70 percent above expected levels.

More recently, however, several meta-analyses of the data (a combination of all previous epidemiological studies) have shown that the risk of developing breast cancer is not all that great (see Table 9). The consensus now is that after fifteen years of estrogen therapy, your risk of developing breast cancer may increase by roughly 30 percent. No studies have shown an increase in deaths from breast cancer among estrogen users, and some have actually shown an increase in the cure rate of breast cancer among women taking postmenopausal hormones. It's not known whether the hormone therapy itself played a role in the higher cure rate or whether the women were screened more diligently, helping to catch their cancers in the early stages, when the cure rate is high.

Among women with a family history of breast cancer, however, those who have ever taken estrogen have a twofold greater risk than those who have never taken it, which is why most women whose mothers or sisters have been diagnosed with breast cancer are often advised *not* to take postmenopausal estrogens.

The exact mechanisms by which estrogen may increase the risk of breast cancer are not known. Estrogen doesn't appear to be an initiator of cancer; that is, it does not turn a normal cell into a cancerous cell. Rather estrogen appears to be a *promoter* of cancer by stimulating cells that have already become cancerous to grow more rapidly.

TABLE 9 — Breast Cancer Risk Associated With Estrogen Use

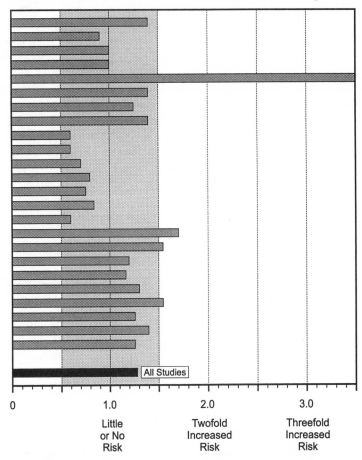

Each bar represents the findings of a single study. Most studies have found little or no increased risk of breast cancer associated with use of postmenopausal estrogens.

More research needs to be conducted before we fully understand the role of postmenopausal hormone therapy in the development of breast cancer. At this point, the benefits to some women, (particularly those at risk of developing heart disease and osteoporosis) clearly outweigh the slightly increased risk of breast cancer. Remember: six times more women die of cardiovascular disease than of breast cancer. Keep in mind, too, that postmenopausal hormone therapy isn't the only possible risk factor for breast cancer: a high-fat diet may contribute to up to 30 percent of breast cancers, and reducing the fat in your diet certainly would be a prudent policy for lowering your risk of breast cancer. Regular exercise also appears to reduce the risk of breast cancer.

Bear in mind that 80 to 90 percent of breast cancers are cured when caught early, which is why close surveillance of all women on hormone therapy is essential. We advise weekly breast self-examination, possibly two breast examinations annually by health care professionals, and most definitely yearly mammograms.

The data on breast cancer risk is not conclusive enough to cause doctors to change the way they prescribe postmenopausal hormones. But studies do point to the need for additional research. Until we know more, it's safe for women who would benefit most from postmenopausal hormones—those with a family history of heart disease, for instance—to take them, provided the women are closely monitored.

Other cancers. What effect do postmenopausal hormones have on your risk of developing other types of cancer? There's some evidence to suggest that postmenopausal estrogens actually may *protect* against fatal colon cancer. In the largest and most recent study, involving more than 400,000 women, those who ever used postmenopausal estrogens had a 29 percent reduction in the risk of developing colon cancer, compared to nonusers. Current users of postmenopausal estrogens had a 45 percent reduction in risk, while those who had used estrogen in the past had a 19 percent reduction in risk. And among women who had been using postmenopausal estrogens for more than ten years and were currently using estrogen, there was a 55 percent reduction in risk. The study volunteers were part of the Cancer Prevention Study II (CPS-II), a large-scale study begun by the American Cancer Society in 1982. The results from the CPS-II study support several other published reports that suggest a protective role of hormones in the development of colorectal cancer.

Although it appears as though postmenopausal estrogens may protect against colorectal cancer, yet another recent study, also based on data from the CPS-II, found the risk of ovarian cancer to be *increased* among long-term users of postmenopausal estrogens. According to this study, involving 240,000 postmenopausal women, the risk of ovarian cancer was 40 percent higher for women who had used postmenopausal estrogens for at least six years and 70 percent higher for women who had used postmenopausal estrogens for at least eleven years, compared to women who had never used postmenopausal estrogens. Past studies investigating an increased risk of ovarian cancer associated with use of postmenopausal estrogens have been inconclusive, however, and the researchers point out that the results of this study should be interpreted with caution. The most important point about this study is that its findings may not apply to women using postmenopausal estrogens today because the normal dose is generally less than that prescribed in the 1970s and 1980s, when women in the study were being treated. In addition, most physicians today prescribe progestogens along with estrogen, which was uncommon in the 1970s and 1980s.

Another consideration to keep in mind is that colon cancer is far more prevalent among women than ovarian cancer. According to the American Cancer Society, an estimated 67,500 women develop colon cancer each year, compared with 26,600 women who develop ovarian cancer. On the other hand, ovarian cancer more often is fatal among women who develop it because it is difficult to detect until it has spread. More than half of all women who develop ovarian cancer die of the disease, compared with about a third of all women who develop colorectal cancer. Remember, too, that heart disease is far more prevalent than either colon or ovarian cancer.

Other complications. One or two studies have shown a slight increase in the risk of developing gallstones among women who take estrogens. However, it's still not clear whether the estrogens actually *caused* the development of gallstones. At any rate, this complication is very rare. If you or your physician suspect you may have gallstones, you may want to undergo an ultrasound scan of your gallbladder before beginning hormone additive therapy.

If you have significant hepatitis or suffered residual liver damage as a result of a past bout with hepatitis, we recommend the use of a patch, pellets, or some other non-oral form of estrogen, which bypasses the liver altogether.

What About Progestogen?

Progestogens are prescribed to prevent overstimulation of the uterine lining by estrogens and hence help protect against the development of endometrial cancer among women who still have an intact uterus. (Women who have had a hysterectomy don't need to take progestogen, even if their ovaries remain intact.) The practice not only prevents endometrial cancer, but also has a protective effect. *Indeed, women who take a progestogen for at least ten days per month have less endometrial cancer than women who take no hormones whatsoever.*

When the practice of prescribing progestogen along with estrogen became more routine in the 1980s, it raised numerous questions about what impact, if any, progestogen would have on the therapeutic effects of estrogen, particularly estrogen's ability to protect against cardiovascular disease. After all, most of the studies on the beneficial effects of postmenopausal hormones involved estrogens alone. The research on progestogen is continuing, but it appears that, in some ways, added progestogen offer some benefits of its own.

Progestogens *do* appear to dampen the effects of estrogens on blood lipids somewhat. However, when progestogens are given cyclically (see pages 164–165) and with intermediate to high doses of estrogens, you'll still experience an *overall increase in cardioprotective factors*, such as HDL cholesterol. One study of women taking estrogen and progestogen showed a 6 percent increase in HDL cholesterol—about half that of women receiving estrogens alone, but still a significant rise. Micronized progesterone appears to have little or no impact on HDL cholesterol, and may be the best choice.

Contrary to popular belief, progestogens have no adverse effect on blood pressure. Again, the idea that progestogens raise blood pressure was based on studies involving the older oral contraceptives, which contained large doses of estrogen and progestogen.

Progestogens don't appear to increase the risk of developing blood clots either. In fact, progestogens may even help prevent blood clots from forming. We found that postmenopausal progestogens *increase* the activity of the anticoagulant plasminogen by 16 to 20 percent. Although we don't yet know what effect these changes have in the body, it's possible that the increased plasminogen may have a protective effect.

Higher blood levels of plasminogen may also help protect against a newly discovered blood lipid, known as apolipoprotein (a), which is thought to take the place of plasminogen in the artery wall and "short-circuit" the blood vessel's natural ability to dissolve clots.

Progestogens *do* increase insulin resistance somewhat, which may be a problem for some women, particularly those with diabetes. Diabetic women who take combination hormones may need to be more closely monitored.

Animal studies have also suggested that progestogens may reduce blood flow. This may somewhat dampen the increase in blood flow associated with estrogens, particularly through the coronary arteries. However, more research needs to be conducted before we know for certain whether the decreased blood flow associated with progestogen leads to an increased risk of heart disease.

In the near future, new types of progestogen and different ways of administering the hormone may be safer still. Preliminary evidence suggests that a new class of synthetic progestogen—*gestodene, desogestrel,* and *norgestimate*—as well as a form of natural micronized oral progesterone, will have little effect on HDL cholesterol in women taking estrogens. A transdermal skin patch containing both estrogen and progestogen may also reduce the negative effects of progestogen on blood lipids because the hormones are absorbed through the skin directly into the bloodstream, instead of passing through the liver (where lipid production and processing occur).

Of course, cardiovascular disease is a result of many different factors, so it's hard to quantify what overall effect progestogens have. Remember, though, that progestogen is needed only if you have an intact uterus, and is prescribed in the lowest possible dose to protect the uterine lining from overstimulation by estrogen. So far, it appears that progestogen doesn't cancel out the good that estrogen does for your heart.

IF YOU TAKE PROGESTOGEN ALONG WITH ESTROGEN, WILL YOU GET MONTHLY PERIODS AGAIN?

This is one of the more pressing questions of women who must take a combination of estrogen and progestogen to protect against endometrial cancer, particularly when the cessation of monthly bleeding is seen as one of the *benefits* of menopause. Indeed, resumption of menstrual-like bleeding is the chief reason women give for *not* taking hormones prescribed to them, or for stopping hormone additive therapy soon after they've begun taking it.

Actually, the bleeding you experience is *not* a real menstrual period in the true sense of the word, since it is the shedding of an artificially stimulated endometrium. *How much* bleeding you expect and *when* you can expect it depends on which one of three estrogen-progestogen regimens you take.

- *Twenty-five-day cyclic regimen.* If you take estrogen for twenty-five days, an added progestogen for days fifteen through twenty-five, followed by five days of no medication, you can expect to experience some bleeding during the five-day interval in which you are taking no hormones.

> ### *If You Take Progestogen Along with Estrogen . . . (Cont.)*
>
> - *Continuous cyclic regimen.* If you take an estrogen every day without a break, along with an added progestogen during the first two weeks of every month, you will experience some bleeding during the middle of the month.
> - *Continuous combined regimen.* If you take an estrogen and progestogen every day, you may experience some irregular bleeding and light spotting for the first four months. (Sixty percent of women on this regimen won't bleed at all during the first four to six months.) After six months, few women will experience any bleeding.
>
> New regimens are now being developed to minimize bleeding even further. One such regimen involves taking estrogen every day, and adding progestogen for fourteen days once every three months. Early studies suggest that this combination protects against endometrial cancer equally well as the three more widely used regimens described above.
>
> For most women the menstrual effects of combined estrogen-progestogen therapy are minimal. A minority of women may experience heavy bleeding, menstrual cramps, and pain that can be relieved with nonsteroidal anti-inflammatory drugs (NSAIDs), such as *ibuprofen* (Advil, Motrin-IB, Nuprin, etc.), *naproxen* (Anaprox, Aleve, Naprosyn), or *mefenamic acid* (Ponstel). Keep in mind, too, that the benefit of taking hormone additive therapy—protection from cardiovascular disease—far outweighs the minor inconvenience of menstrual-like bleeding.

What About Androgens?

Although testosterone and other androgens are considered "male" reproductive hormones, women produce a certain amount of androgens, too. Prescription androgens are occasionally used to help alleviate severe menopausal symptoms. Preliminary evidence suggests that androgens given to menopausal women contribute to an increased sense of well-being, improved sex drive, fewer headaches, relief from depression, and increased bone mass. But what effect do androgens have on a woman's risk of developing cardiovascular disease?

While some researchers worried that giving androgens to women would raise their blood cholesterol levels, to date most studies involving estrogen combined with a non-oral androgen have found little or no change in blood lipids. However, oral androgens may reduce levels of protective high-density lipoproteins.

On the other hand, oral androgens appear to lower blood triglycerides, and may help offset the *rise* in blood triglycerides often triggered by oral estrogens. In a recent study we conducted, women taking an oral estrogen-androgen combination experienced a 20 percent decrease in blood triglycerides. So there may actually be a role for androgens in the prevention of cardiovascular disease.

Who Should Not Take Hormones?

The list of women who *should not* take hormones is actually quite small. If you have unexplained vaginal bleeding, estrogen-dependent breast cancer, or have had a recent heart attack, you definitely should *not* take hormones.

Although in the past, all women who had had endometrial cancer (cancer of the lining of the uterus) were advised not to take estrogen, the issue is being reevaluated, and, under certain circumstances, some women with a history of endometrial cancer may be able to take estrogen safely. Women with a history of cervical cancer and certain types of ovarian cancer may also be able to take estrogen; ask your doctor.

It is still not certain whether or not estrogen encourages the growth of melanoma, the most deadly form of skin cancer. Past studies have found estrogen receptors in melanomas, suggesting that estrogen may help fuel the cancer's spread. More recent studies have suggested that the cancer isn't influenced by estrogen in any way. If you have had a melanoma, discuss with your doctor whether or not you should take estrogen.

Some women will need to be monitored more closely while taking hormone therapy, including women with a family history of breast cancer, those with seizure disorders, hypertension, fibroid tumors of the uterus, high blood cholesterol, migraine headaches, previous superficial blood clots in the legs (thrombophlebitis), endometriosis, and gallbladder disease.

Heavy smokers, on the other hand, should not take estrogen; smokers who need estrogen therapy should stop smoking before starting therapy.

Should You Take Postmenopausal Estrogens?

When considering whether to take hormone additive therapy to help protect against cardiovascular disease, you and your physician should consider whether you have any of the following risk factors:

1. A family history of premature heart disease (that is, if your father or a brother suffered *angina* (chest pain), a heart attack, or sudden death before age fifty-five OR your mother or a sister developed heart disease before age sixty)
2. Parents or brothers or sisters with elevated blood cholesterol levels
3. A parent or sibling with high blood pressure or diabetes
4. Elevated blood pressure and cholesterol levels (total cholesterol above 240 mg/dl of blood, LDL cholesterol above 140 mg/dl, triglycerides above 300 mg/dl, or HDL cholesterol below 35 mg/dl)
5. An early menopause (before age forty)

If you have one or more of the above risk factors, you should seriously consider using estrogen as added protection against heart disease in your postmenopausal years.

If You Decide to Use Estrogen

Once you have made the decision to protect yourself against heart disease with postmenopausal estrogen preparations, you will have to work with your physician to determine which form of hormone therapy is best for you.

Estrogen is usually given orally in tablet form, but it can also be administered by patch, injection, or pellet implantation (into the fatty tissue under the skin, usually in the lower abdomen above the groin or in the upper buttocks). See "Postmenopausal Estrogen Preparations" on page 170. Vaginal estrogen creams, which are usually prescribed to relieve postmenopausal vaginal dryness, generally are not recommended for the prevention of cardiovascular disease because, when used in low doses as directed by your physician, these forms of estrogen don't raise blood levels of estrogen high enough to provide protection.

Different types and amounts of estrogen may affect you in different ways. For instance, oral estrogens raise levels of protective HDL cholesterol. Unfortunately oral estrogens also raise blood triglyceride levels, and may not be appropriate for women with high triglycerides. On the other hand, the estrogen patch doesn't raise triglycerides, but it also doesn't raise HDL cholesterol. Here are some general guidelines that you can use in your discussion with your physician:

If you have high blood pressure: As we mentioned earlier, oral estrogens actually *lower* blood pressure. For the minority of women whose blood pressure rises after beginning hormonal therapy, or for women whose hypertension is related to the hormone *renin*, the estrogen patch should be used.

If you have diabetes: If your blood triglycerides are elevated, you should use the patch, since oral estrogens have been associated with an increase in blood triglycerides. If your levels of HDL cholesterol are not too low, you could also consider using an oral estrogen-androgen combination, since the androgens appear to offset the rise in blood triglycerides associated with oral estrogens. Otherwise, oral estrogens are fine because they actually *lower* blood sugar levels.

If you have a history of blood clots: Women with previous deep venous thrombosis *can* take estrogen therapy, particularly if the blood clot was from a nonrecurring cause. (For instance, a woman who developed phlebitis after a cesarean section twenty years ago can safely use hormone therapy.)

What kind of estrogen is best? If you have a remote deep venous thrombosis, the type of estrogen you take makes no difference. If you have recently developed a blood clot from a nonrecurring cause (for instance, after a hysterectomy), you should use the skin patch, which has less of an effect on coagulation factors produced by the liver.

Should you stop estrogen therapy before surgery? It's probably not necessary, but it may be prudent to do so for one month prior to surgery. Immediately after surgery, you should use the skin patch.

A precautionary note: All women with a history of blood clots should be closely monitored. Your physician can test for levels of fibrinogen, anticoagulants (such as antithrombin III activity), and the overall marker of the clotting mechanism—prothrombin time. We advocate the use of a junior aspirin (60 milligrams) every third day. Aspirin helps decrease platelet adhesiveness and encourages dilation of the blood vessels. (Note: You should take aspirin regularly only while under a doctor's supervision; see page 178.) You should also exercise, which increases blood flow through your body and may raise levels of certain anticoagulants. Moreover, *you should not smoke*. Cigarette smoking increases the "stickiness" of blood platelets, decreasing clotting time, increasing blood thickness, and increasing the likelihood that a blood clot will form. Plus, cigarette smoking appears to damage the lining of the arteries and depresses the production of the anticoagulant prostacyclin by the blood vessel wall, both of which may increase the risk that a blood clot will form.

POSTMENOPAUSAL HORMONE PREPARATIONS

Brand name	Type of Estrogen	Available Dosages	Manufacturer
ORAL ESTROGENS			
Premarin	Conjugated equine estrogens	0.3 mg 0.625 mg 0.9 mg 1.25 mg 2.5 mg	Wyeth-Ayerst
Estrace	Micronized estradiol	1.0 mg 2.0 mg	Mead Johnson
Estratab	Esterified estrogens	0.3 mg 0.625 mg 1.25 mg 2.5 mg	Solvay
Menest	Esterified estrogens	0.3 mg 0.625 mg 1.25 mg 2.5 mg	SmithKline Beecham
Ogen	Estropipate	0.625 mg 1.25 mg 2.5 mg 5.0 mg	Abbott
VAGINAL ESTROGEN CREAMS			
Premarin	Conjugated equine estrogens	0.625 mg	Wyeth-Ayerst
Estrace	17beta-estradiol	0.1 mg	Mead Johnson
Ogen	Estropipate	1.5 mg	Abbott
Ortho Dienestrol	Dienestrol	0.01%	Ortho
Estragard	Dienestrol	0.01%	Solvay
Diethylstilbestrol suppositories	Diethylstilbestrol	0.1 mg 0.5 mg	Lilly
PARENTERAL ESTROGENS (INJECTIONS, PELLETS, PATCHES)			
Depo-estradiol	Estradiol cypionate	1 mg	Upjohn
Delestrogen	Estradiol valerate	10 mg 20 mg 40 mg	Squibb

Brand name	Type of Estrogen	Available Dosages	Manufacturer
Estravel	Estradiol valerate	10 mg 20 mg	Solvay
Estrapel	Estradiol pellet	25 mg/pellet	Bartor
Estraderm	Transdermal estradiol	0.05 mg/day 0.1 mg/day	Ciba-Geigy
Climara	Transdermal estradiol	0.05 mg/day 0.1 mg/day	Berlex
PROGESTOGENS			
Amen	Medroxyprogesterone acetate	10 mg	Carnick
Aygestin	Norethindrone acetate	5 mg	Wyeth-Ayerst
Curretab	Medroxyprogesterone acetate	10 mg	Solvay
Cycrin	Medroxyprogesterone acetate	10 mg	Wyeth-Ayerst
Norlutate	Norethindrone acetate	5 mg	Parke-Davis
Norlutin	Norethindrone	5 mg	Parke-Davis
Megace	Megesterol acetate	20 mg 40 mg	Bristol-Myers
Ovrette	Norgestrel	0.075 mg	Wyeth-Ayerst
Micronor	Norethindrone	0.35 mg	Ortho
	Micronized oral progesterone	100 mg	
Provera	Medroxyprogesterone acetate	10 mg	Upjohn
	Progesterone vaginal suppositories	25 mg 50 mg	
ESTROGEN-PROGESTOGEN COMBINATIONS			
Prempro	Conjugated equine estrogens and medroxyprogesterone acetate	0.625 mg 2.5 mg	Wyeth-Ayerst
Premphase	Conjugated equine estrogens and medroxyprogesterone acetate	0.625 mg 5.0 mg	Wyeth-Ayerst

POSTMENOPAUSAL HORMONE PREPARATIONS

Brand name	Type of Estrogen	Available Dosages	Manufacturer
ORAL ANDROGENS			
Oreton	Methyltestosterone	5 mg	Schering
Metandren	Methyltestosterone	5 mg	Ciba
Halotestin	Fluoxymesterone	5 mg	Upjohn
Fluoxy-mesterone	Fluoxymesterone	5 mg	Solvay
Ora-Testryl	Fluoxymesterone	5 mg	Squibb
Testred	Methyltestosterone	10 mg	ICN
INJECTABLE ANDROGENS			
Depo-testosterone	Testosterone cypionate	50 mg/ml	Upjohn
Delatestryl	Testosterone enanthate	100 mg/ml	Squibb
Durabolin	Nandrolone phenpropionate	25 to 50 mg/ml wkly	Organon
Deca-Durabolin	Nandrolone decanoate	50 to 100 mg/ml wkly	Organon
ANDROGEN PELLETS			
Testopel	Testosterone	75 mg	Bartor
ANDROGEN OINTMENTS			
	Testosterone proprianate	2% in a petrolatum base	
ESTROGEN-ANDROGEN COMBINATIONS			
Estratest tablets	Esterified estrogens Methyltestosterone	1.25 mg 2.5 mg	Solvay
Estratest H.S. tablets	Esterified estrogens Methyltestosterone	0.625 mg 1.25 mg	Solvay
Premarin with methyl-testosterone	Conjugated equine estrogens Methyltestosterone	0.625 mg 1.25 mg 5 mg 10 mg	Wyeth-Ayerst
Depo-Testadiol	Estradiol cypionate Testosterone cypionate	2 mg 50 mg	Upjohn

If you have high blood cholesterol and/or a family history of cardio-vascular disease: Most of the studies showing a protective effect are based on the use of conjugated oral estrogens (specifically Premarin). We found that Ogen (estropipate) was also highly effective in reducing blood cholesterol, especially among women with elevated cholesterol (above 260 mg/dl). After twelve months, total cholesterol of the women taking Ogen in our study fell 3.4 percent, LDL cholesterol dropped 8.3 percent, and HDL cholesterol rose 9.7 percent. If you have high cholesterol and decreased HDL cholesterol, you can take oral Premarin, Ogen, Estrace, or other equivalents.

If your triglycerides are elevated, however, the patch may be a better choice, because oral estrogens may raise triglycerides. (If you have elevated triglycerides *and* fairly high levels of HDL cholesterol, your physician may recommend an estrogen-androgen combination. Oral androgens have been found to lower triglycerides.)

As for progestogens, very low doses of *19-nortestosterone* or *micronized progesterone* are preferable because they have been shown to have the least effect on blood lipids. You should take the minimum dose needed to protect against endometrial cancer. You should also take a *cyclic* rather than a *continuous* regimen of progestogens, since this further limits the amount of time you are exposed to progestogens.

(Note: The transdermal estrogen patch also alters blood lipids, but usually only after four to six months of treatment. The main positive effect of the patch is to lower LDL cholesterol levels, rather than increasing protective HDL cholesterol levels. So if your HDL levels are low, in our opinion you must use oral estrogens.)

If you have established coronary heart disease: Hormonal therapy also appears to be useful in women with established coronary heart disease. Studies have shown that estrogen-users who have balloon angioplasty or bypass surgery live longer than those who don't take estrogen. And since estrogens work so well at raising HDL cholesterol and lowering LDL cholesterol, they can be used for the treatment of patients with high blood cholesterol (*hypercholesterolemia*). Of course, if you have high cholesterol levels, you should also eat a low-fat diet and exercise regularly. You may also need to take specific cholesterol-lowering drugs (see Chapter 10).

Before beginning hormone therapy, you should have a complete physical, including Pap smear, pelvic and breast examination, and a mammogram (low-dose X ray of the breasts). You should undergo these examinations once a year while you are using estrogen. Check your breasts at home *once a week* ("always on Sundays"); this way, you'll get into the habit of examining your breasts on a regular basis. You will also become more familiar with your breasts, and will be better able to detect any *unfamiliar* lumps.

After beginning hormone therapy, your blood cholesterol levels should be monitored periodically (every two years if cholesterol levels are normal, and once every six months if they're elevated) to ensure that the therapy is effective. Again, we recommend you undergo a complete lipid profile rather than just have your total cholesterol levels measured. The lipid profile gives your doctor a better idea of how well the hormone therapy is working. You should also keep in mind that hormone therapy works best when used in conjunction with other preventive measures, such as a low-fat diet and exercise.

If You Cannot or Decide Not to Take Estrogen

If you are one of the few women who has been advised *not* to take estrogen because of a family history of breast cancer or other problem, or if you simply choose not to take estrogen during your postmenopausal years, you can still protect yourself against coronary heart disease. You should at the very least be certain to eat a diet low in fat and cholesterol, get plenty of exercise, and follow the other guidelines outlined in the previous chapters for lowering your risk. If your blood cholesterol levels are high, lipid-lowering medications, discussed in the next chapter, are another option.

CHAPTER 10

Drugs Used to Prevent Coronary Artery Disease

IF DIET, EXERCISE, and other lifestyle changes aren't effective in lowering your cholesterol, your physician has an arsenal of highly effective drugs to help do the job.

Remember, though, that *all* drugs carry some risk, and most drugs work best when used *in conjunction with* the lifestyle measures we've outlined in previous chapters.

Lipid-lowering Drugs

The most widely prescribed lipid-lowering drugs can reduce LDL cholesterol by an average of 25 to 30 percent *when used in conjunction with a low-cholesterol, low-fat diet.* What's more, recent studies have found that some of the newer lipid-lowering medications not only lower blood cholesterol, but also promote the regression of artery-narrowing plaques. In addition, these drugs have been shown to improve the ability of the endothelium (the innermost lining of the artery) to function normally. So in effect, lipid-lowering medications help protect against further damage from heart disease in a number of important ways.

Lipid-lowering medications are generally recommended to women with LDL cholesterol levels above 190 mg/dl that have failed to respond to at least six months of diet therapy. Women with two or more risk factors for coronary artery disease along with LDL cholesterol above 160 mg/dl may also be considered for drug therapy if dietary measures don't help.

Triglyceride-lowering drugs may be recommended if you have high triglycerides (above 250 mg/dl) along with high LDL cholesterol or low HDL cholesterol, if you have very high triglycerides (over 1,000 mg/dl), or if you have a personal or family history of coronary heart disease.

The following drugs are commonly prescribed to lower elevated LDL cholesterol levels. Some have the added benefit of raising HDL cholesterol and may also be recommended for women with low HDL cholesterol levels.

Bile Acid Sequestrants
The two sequestrants available today, *cholestyramine* (brand names Choly-bar, Questran, Questran Light) and *colestipol* (brand names Colestid, Cholestabyl) indirectly lower LDL cholesterol by preventing bile acids in the intestine from circulating in the bloodstream.

The drugs, which come in powder form and must be mixed with water or fruit juice, lower LDL cholesterol from 15 to 30 percent without affecting HDL cholesterol. Side effects include constipation, bloating, nausea, and gas.

Niacin
A prescription form of the water-soluble B-vitamin niacin (also known as nicotinic acid) has been used safely to lower blood cholesterol for more than thirty years. Niacin decreases the liver's production of VLDL cholesterol, which in turn lowers LDL cholesterol in the bloodstream. Niacin also raises HDL cholesterol.

The biggest drawback to niacin is that it causes a number of bothersome side effects, including *flushing* (reddening of the skin and heat sensations), elevated levels of blood sugar and *uric acid* (a byproduct of protein metabolism; high levels can lead to *gout*), nausea, diarrhea, heart palpitations, and liver toxicity. For these reasons, you should take niacin *only* under a doctor's supervision. Taking niacin with meals or taking aspirin or a nonsteroidal anti-inflammatory drug (such as ibuprofen) an hour or so before taking niacin reduces flushes.

Niacin is sold under the following brand names: Endur-Acin, Nia-Bid, Niac, Niacels, Nico-400, Nicobid Tempules, Nicolar, Nicotinex Elixir, Slo-Niacin, Span-Niacin, and Tega-Span.

Statins
These drugs lower blood cholesterol by inhibiting the liver enzyme *HMGCoA reductase*, which regulates the liver's production of cholesterol. *Lovastatin* (brand name Mevacor) reduces LDL cholesterol by 25 to 45 percent. Two

other drugs, *simvastatin* (Zocor) and *pravastatin* (Pravachol) have a similar track record.

Side effects include constipation, diarrhea, upset stomach, gas, headache, skin rash, and muscle weakness. But these are uncommon, occurring in only about 5 percent of patients who take the drug. Long-term side effects, if any, aren't known.

Fibric Acids

These drugs, including *gemfibrozil* (brand name Lopid) and *clofibrate* (brand names Abitrate, Atromid-S), are primarily used to reduce the risk of *pancreatitis* (inflammation of the pancreas) among people with high blood triglycerides. But gemfibrozil has been shown to reduce the risk of coronary heart disease as well—at least in men. Gemfibrozil lowers triglycerides and raises HDL cholesterol.

Stomach upset, abdominal pain, and other gastrointestinal symptoms are common side effects.

Probucol

This drug moderately lowers LDL cholesterol, although no one's sure exactly how it works. Probucol (brand name Lorelco) also lowers HDL cholesterol, so it is generally not recommended unless other cholesterol-lowering medications are ineffective. Probucol is a powerful antioxidant, however, and may protect against harmful oxidation of LDL cholesterol.

Psyllium Seed

When combined with a low-fat, low-cholesterol diet, psyllium seed, a soluble fiber found in some foods and in bulk fiber laxatives such as Metamucil, has been found to be quite effective in lowering LDL cholesterol without affecting HDL cholesterol. In one of the best-designed studies to date, by researchers at the University of Minnesota, volunteers who took 3.4 grams of psyllium seed (1 teaspoon) three times a day lowered total cholesterol an additional 4.8 percent and lowered LDL cholesterol an additional 8.2 percent beyond the cholesterol-lowering effects of their low-fat diet. University of Kentucky physician James W. Anderson has reported up to a 14.8 percent decline in total cholesterol and a 20.2 percent decline in LDL cholesterol among the hypercholesterolemic men he treated.

No one's sure exactly how psyllium works, although we suspect that psyllium somehow slows the amount of cholesterol or fatty acids absorbed by the intestine.

Side effects, including abdominal cramping and fullness, bloating, and gas, are minor and usually don't last long.

Some breakfast cereals now contain psyllium seed, but one of the best sources of this soluble fiber is over-the-counter bulk fiber laxatives, such as Metamucil. (Generic brands are also available.) Metamucil now comes in the form of convenient wafers, too. If you have high cholesterol, you may want to ask your physician about supplementing your low-fat diet with psyllium.

Antithrombic Drugs

These drugs don't affect blood cholesterol. Rather, they protect by help-ing to prevent the development of blood clots that could trigger a heart attack or stroke. There are actually three types of antithrombic drugs: *antiplatelets*, such as aspirin, reduce the stickiness of platelets, helping to prevent the formation of a blood clot. *Anticoagulants*, such as heparin and warfarin, also prevent blood clots from forming but in a different way: these drugs slow down the clotting action of blood by inactivating or interfering with numerous coagulants in the blood and produced by the liver.

The third type of antithrombic drugs are known as *thrombolytic* or *fibrinolytic* drugs. These drugs dissolve existing blood clots by increasing the blood level and action of *plasmin*, an enzyme that breaks up the tough fibrin strands that hold a clot together. Thrombolytic and fibrinolytic drugs are generally used for treating a heart attack or stroke, not for preventing one. (For more on these drugs, see Chapter 12.)

Aspirin and Other Antiplatelet Drugs

One way of reducing your risk of a life-threatening blood clot is as close as your home medicine cabinet. Aspirin is a powerful antiplatelet drug that works by tipping the balance between the substance prostacyclin, which helps prevent the formation of blood clots, and thromboxane, which promotes the development of clots, so that prostacyclin gets the upper hand. When you take aspirin, it suppresses the production of both prostacyclin in the blood vessel wall and thromboxane, manufactured by blood platelets. But aspirin's effects on prostacyclin last for only six hours, while aspirin suppresses thromboxane for three days. As a result, when you take aspirin regularly, your blood becomes more resistant to forming a clot.

A few major studies—all involving men—suggest that taking aspirin reduces the risk of heart attacks and strokes caused by blood clots (thrombosis). However, aspirin-takers in the studies suffered more strokes from cerebral hemorrhage than those who took a placebo.

The Nurse's Health Study, involving more than 40,000 female nurses, also found beneficial effects of aspirin. Women who took between one and six aspirin a week registered a 25 percent reduction in the risk of having a heart attack. Women over age fifty and those at high risk of developing coronary heart disease had the greatest reduction in risk. Women who took seven or more aspirin per week, however, didn't enjoy any greater protection, and those who took fifteen or more aspirin per week were at a greater risk of suffering a cerebral hemorrhage.

Definitive results on the benefit of taking aspirin to women won't be known until the results of the Women's Health Study are tallied in 1997. This is a large study of low-dose aspirin use among more than 40,000 female nurses age forty-five and over.

Your doctor may recommend that you use aspirin if you already have coronary artery disease and are at a greater risk of having a heart attack or stroke, and after heart and blood vessel surgery.

Although aspirin is readily available over the counter and without a prescription, you should not regularly take aspirin to prevent a heart attack or stroke without first discussing it with your doctor. If you have liver or kidney disease, a peptic ulcer, gastrointestinal bleeding, or other bleeding problems, you may not be able to take aspirin at all, or you may need to adjust the amount you take. Since aspirin prolongs bleeding, you should notify your physician that you're taking aspirin if you're scheduled for any kind of surgery. Also, if you have uncontrolled hypertension or any condition that might increase the risk of a stroke, you should not take aspirin routinely without first checking with your physician. When we prescribe aspirin to patients in our clinic, we recommend taking a junior aspirin (60 milligrams) every three days.

Other antiplatelet drugs available by prescription are dipyridamole (Persantine), sulfinpyrazone (Anturane), and ticlopidine (Ticlid).

Anticoagulants

The anticoagulants heparin and warfarin are generally prescribed to prevent clots from forming after a heart attack. You may also have to take one of these anticoagulants if you have a type of arrhythmia known as *atrial fibrillation*, or if you have an artificial heart valve. Both of these heart conditions predispose you to the development of blood clots.

Heparin is given by injection and is effective immediately upon entering the bloodstream. Warfarin is given in the form of a pill and takes a few days to become effective.

Side effects of both heparin and warfarin include internal bleeding, especially in the gastrointestinal tract or kidney, and easy bruisability.

CHAPTER 11

If You Already Have Coronary Artery Disease

IF YOU HAVE already been diagnosed with coronary artery disease, there is plenty you and your doctor can do to reduce your risk of having a heart attack. These include the use of numerous medications, angioplasty, or bypass surgery, all of which, in their own way, help to compensate for the blockages in the coronary arteries and maintain a steady blood supply to the heart. Each has its own benefits and risks.

There's also evidence that making lifestyle changes alone—changing the way you eat, exercise, and cope with stress—can sometimes prevent a heart attack and reverse the narrowing of the arteries that has already occurred. But even this option, like the others, may not be suitable for everyone.

No matter what treatment you and your physician choose, lifestyle changes and risk-reducing strategies, such as following a low-fat diet, exercising regularly, and reducing stress, should be an integral part of your treatment plan.

You and your doctor, working together, will have to determine what treatment or combination of treatments is best for you. For your part, this means learning as much as you can about the benefits and risks of each treatment option so that you can make an informed decision. That's the subject of this chapter.

Drug Therapy

Various medications have proven to be highly effective in treating existing heart disease. (See Figure 10 on page 183.) The advantages of using drug therapies are that medications are noninvasive and therefore are much less risky than surgical procedures. They're less expensive than surgery too. The disadvantages: all drugs have side effects, and you may have to try more than one medication to find one that's best suited to your needs. And while drugs *are* less expensive than surgery, they, too, cost money. Still, for women with early stage coronary artery disease, and for those with such an extensive accumulation of plaques that surgery cannot adequately address the problem, drug therapy (combined with an aggressive risk-reducing strategy) may be one of the best options.

If you have high blood cholesterol, your physician will likely recommend that you use one of the cholesterol-lowering medications discussed in Chapter 10. If you have angina or silent ischemia (reduced blood flow to the heart that doesn't cause any pain), your doctor may prescribe one or more of the following medications as well:

Beta-Blockers
These drugs, given in the form of a pill, block parts of the sympathetic nervous system, reducing the workload of the heart by lowering the heart rate and relaxing the blood vessel walls. Some beta-blockers also help dilate the blood vessels.

The downside of these drugs is that angina may worsen if the medication is stopped. In addition, beta-blockers may aggravate angina if you also have coronary spasms. Because these drugs may cause or aggravate asthma or bronchospasms, they should not be used by people with either of these medical conditions. You may also experience a decreased tolerance to exercise while taking these drugs. Some people may experience depression, chronic fatigue, and lethargy. Also, if you have insulin-dependent diabetes, you may not be able to take beta-blockers because they can mask insulin reactions.

Nitrates
These drugs (also known as nitroglycerine) dilate the coronary arteries directly, which increases blood flow to the heart. Nitrates also reduce the workload of the heart by dilating the veins, which slows the return of blood to the heart for oxygenation.

Nitroglycerine is administered in several ways. Sometimes, if you have severe angina, your physician may prescribe a tablet that you can slip under your tongue for relief from pain within a few minutes. Nitroglycerine also comes in capsules and as a transdermal patch for daily use. In addition, this medication may be administered by constant infusion via a pump.

One of the most bothersome side effects associated with the use of nitroglycerine is *orthostatic hypotension*, a sudden drop in blood pressure

FIGURE 10 — Drugs Commonly Used to Treat Heart Disease

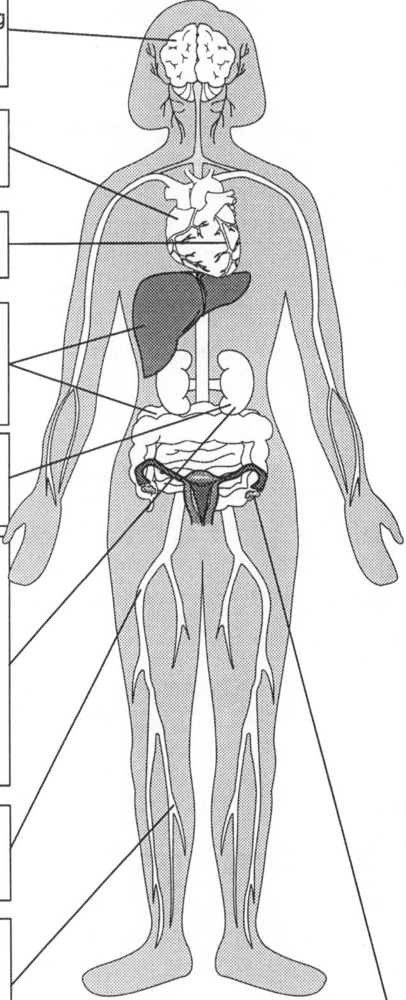

Beta-blockers affect parts of the sympathetic nervous system, slowing the heart rate and reducing the contracting power of the heart.

Antiarrhythmics alter the conduction of electrical signals in the heart to help restore normal rhythm.

Nitrates dilate the coronary arteries to increase blood flow to the heart.

Lipid Lowering Drugs either decrease absorption of cholesterol from the intestines or interfere with the liver's production of cholesterol and triglycerides.

Diuretics increase the excretion of sodium and water from the kidneys, reducing blood pressure.

Ace Inhibitors interfere with production of an enzyme (angiotensin converting enzyme, or ACE) needed to help convert the kidney enzyme *renin* into *angiotensin*, a powerful blood vessel constrictor. Thus, the drugs relax and open the blood vessels, lowering blood pressure and reducing the heart's workload.

Calcium Channel Blockers interfere with the entry of calcium into the blood vessel walls, helping to relax and dilate the arteries.

Antithrombic Drugs either prevent the development of blood clots or help to break up existing blood clots by interfering with various stages of the formation of blood clots.

Postmenopausal Estrogens lower harmful LDL cholesterol and raise protective HDL cholesterol; reduce the stickiness of platelets, helping to prevent the formation of blood clots; and relax the blood vessels, encouraging increased blood flow through the arteries and possibly lowering blood pressure.

when you sit or stand up quickly. In fact, if you already have low blood pressure (a systolic pressure below 90 mmHg), you *should not* use nitroglycerine. Other side effects include headache, dizziness, and flushing, a rapid heart beat (tachycardia) and, rarely, skin rash.

Calcium Channel Blockers

These drugs block or interfere with the transport of calcium in muscle tissue, nerve tissue, and blood vessel walls. As a result, they slow the spread of electrical activity through the heart's conduction system, reducing the heart's rate and contractility. Calcium channel blockers also relax the artery walls. In these ways, calcium channel blockers lower the heart's workload and enhance blood flow through the coronary arteries. (Calcium channel blockers are prescribed to lower blood pressure and treat arrhythmias as well.)

Side effects include low blood pressure, heart rhythm disturbances, fluid retention, confusion and dizziness, and constipation.

Antiarrhythmics

These drugs, such as digitalis (Digoxin), disopyramide (Napamide, Norpace Norpace CR), procainamide (Procan SR, Promine, Pronestyl, Rhythmin), and quinidine (Cardioquin, Cinquin, Duraquin, Quinaglute, Quinora), help regulate the heart's rhythm by altering the patterns of electrical conduction within the heart. (These drugs are discussed in more detail in Chapter 15.)

Postmenopausal Estrogens

Numerous studies have found that postmenopausal estrogens can help prevent coronary artery disease. There's some evidence to suggest that women with coronary artery disease can benefit from estrogen too. In one study involving 2,268 postmenopausal women undergoing coronary angiography, those who had received estrogen lived longer after the procedure than those who did not. Among women with mild to moderate narrowing of the arteries, the ten-year survival was 95.6 percent in women who had ever used estrogen, compared to 85 percent in women who had never used estrogen. In women with moderate to severe coronary artery disease, survival was 97 percent among "ever users," compared with 60 percent among "never users."

In another study, women who took estrogen after undergoing coronary artery bypass surgery fared better than nonusers. In that study, involving 943 women who had bypass surgery from 1972 to 1985, five-year survival for those who used estrogen was 98 percent, compared with 81 percent for nonusers. Ten-year survival was 69 percent for estrogen users, compared with 46 percent for nonusers.

More research needs to be conducted before estrogen can be routinely prescribed as part of a treatment regimen for women with coronary artery disease, but, so far, it appears that estrogen won't worsen your condition and may even help. (For a complete discussion on the benefits and risks of estrogen, see Chapter 9.)

Aspirin and Other Anticoagulants

If you have unstable angina, you may be prescribed aspirin in addition to antiangina medications. Aspirin helps prevent the formation of blood clots on existing plaques, thus reducing the risk of a heart attack.

Aspirin is the least expensive and most widely available drug used to help prevent blood clots, but other prescription medications are available, as well. These include heparin, a drug that must be administered by injection and is usually given for only a few days at a time; and warfarin, a drug in the form of a pill that must be taken for several days before it becomes effective.

TREATMENT STRATEGIES FOR MICROVASCULAR ANGINA

If you have chest pain with no evidence of coronary artery disease, some of the drugs normally used to treat angina may not always bring relief. What kind of treatment regimen can you expect?

If an exercise stress test reveals that blood flow to the heart is, in fact, reduced during strenuous activity, your physician may recommend that you be treated with antianginal medications, including nitrates and calcium channel blockers. Postmenopausal estrogens, particularly non-oral types, such as the transdermal estrogen patch, can be highly effective. If these drugs don't work, your doctor will likely continue looking for other causes of the chest pain.

In the meantime, you can take some comfort in knowing that the pain is *not* life threatening. In addition, there's no need to limit your normal activity or to stop exercising. (In fact, you will be encouraged to continue exercising.) You should also be aware that the use of narcotics to treat this kind of chest pain is not recommended. And repeat hospitalizations and cardiac catheterizations are neither useful nor necessary.

SOME COMMONLY PRESCRIBED CARDIAC MEDICATIONS

Type of Drug	Prescribed for	How It Works	Potential Side Effects
BETA-BLOCKERS			
Acebutolol (Sectral)	Angina,	These drugs	Fatigue, lethargy,
Atenolol (Tenormin)	hypertension	block specific	depression,
Betaxolol (Kerlone)	arrhythmias.	actions of the	impotence,
Carteolol (Cartrol)	(May also be	sympathetic	increased blood
Labetalol (Normodyne,	prescribed for	nervous system,	lipid and/or uric
Trandate)	mitral valve	decreasing the	acid levels,
Metoprolol (Lopressor,	prolapse and	contracting	decreased exercise
Toprol XL)	numerous non-	power of the	tolerance,
Nadolol (Corgard)	cardiac	heart. Some beta-	possible
Penbutolol (Levatol)	conditions, such	blockers also slow	worsening of
Pindolol (Visken)	as migraine	the heart rate.	angina after
Propranolol (Inderal,	headaches and		medication is
Ipran)	hyperthyroidism.)		stopped.
Timolol (Blocadren)			
CALCIUM CHANNEL BLOCKERS			
Bepridil (Vascor)	Angina,	These drugs	Headache, water
Diltiazem (Cardizem	hypertension,	interfere with the	retention, heart
Dilacor)	arrhythmias.	entry of calcium	rhythm
Felodipine (Plendil)		into muscle tissue	disturbances,
Isradipine (DynaCirc)		and blood vessel	constipation.
Nicardipine (Cardene)		walls, helping to	
Nifedipine (Adalat,		relax and dilate	
Procardia)		the arteries.	
Nimodipine (Nimotop)			
Verapamil (Calan,			
Isoptin, Verelan)			

Type of Drug	Prescribed for	How It Works	Potential Side Effects
NITRATES			
Nitroglycerin (Nitrogard, Nitrospray, Nitrostat)	Angina, and during recovery after a heart attack.	These drugs dilate the coronary arteries to increase blood flow to the heart muscle.	Orthostatic hypotention (a drop in blood pressure upon standing), headache, dizziness, flushing, rapid heartbeat.
Long-acting nitroglycerin (Nitro-Bid, Nitroglyn, Nitrong, Nitrospan, Nitrostat)			
Nitroglycerin patches (Deponit, Minitran, Nitrocine, Nitrodisc, NTG-5, NTG-15, Nitro-Dur, Trans-derm-Nitro)			
Isosorbide dinitrate (Dilatrate, Iso-Bid, Isordil, Onset-5, Sorate, Sorbitrate)			
Erythrityl tetranitrate (Cardilate)			
Penaerythritol tetranitrate (Cardilate)			
Pentaerythritol tetranitrate (Dilar, Duotrate, Naptrate, Pentritol, Pentylan, Peritrate, PETN)			
2 percent nitroglycerine ointment (Nitro-Bid, Nitrol, Nitrong, Nitrostat)			
Isosorbide Mononitrate (Ismo, Monoket, Imdur)			

Type of Drug	Prescribed for	How It Works	Potential Side Effects
ANTIARRHYTHMIC DRUGS			
Adenosine (Adenocard I.V.)	Abnormal heart rhythms	These drugs restore normal heart rhythms by altering the conduction of electrical signals in the heart.	Possible worsening of arrhythmias, nausea, vomiting, diarrhea, confusion, sedation, dizziness.
Atropine (Atropine)			
Digitoxin (Crystodigin)			
Digoxin (Lanoxin, Lanoxicaps)			
Disopyramide (Napamide, Norpace)			
Encainide (Enkaid)			
Flecainide (Tambocor)			
Indecainide (Decabid)			
Lidocaine (Xylocaine)			
Mexiletine (Mexitil)			
Morizicine (Ethmozine)			
Phenytoin (Dilantin)			
Procainamide (Procan, Promine, Pronestyl, Rhythmin)			
Propafenone (Rhythmol)			
Quinidine (Cardioquin, Cinquin, Duraquin, Quinaglute, Quinalan, Quine, Quinidex, Quinora)			
ANTIPLATELET DRUGS			
Aspirin	Prevention of heart attack or stroke.	These drugs reduce the stickiness of platelets, helping to prevent the development of blood clots.	Stomach irritation, ringing in the ears, hearing loss, mild indigestion.
Dipyridamole (Persantine)			
Sulfinpyrazone (Anturane)			
Ticlopidine (Ticlid)			
ANTICOAGULANT DRUGS			
Enoxaparin (Lovenox)	Prevention of clots caused by heart attacks, atrial fibrillation, and artificial heart valves.	These drugs slow the clotting action of the blood.	Internal bleeding, bruising.
Heparin-Calcium (Calciparine)			
Heparin-Sodium (Liquaemin)			
Warfarin (Coumadin, Panwarfin)			

Type of Drug	Prescribed for	How It Works	Potential Side Effects
THROMBOLYTIC DRUGS			
Streptokinase (KabiKinase, Streptase) Tissue-Plasminogen Activator (tPA) (Activase) Urokinase (Abbokinase, Win-Kinase) Anistreplase (Eminase)	To dissolve blood clots while a heart attack is in progress.	These drugs dissolve the tough fibrin strands that hold blood clots together.	Allergic reaction, increased risk of bleeding and bruising.
ANGIOTENSIN-CONVERTING ENZYME (ACE) INHIBITORS			
Benazepril (Lotensin) Captopril (Capoten) Enalapril (Vasotec) Enalaprilat (Vasotec I.V.) Fosinopril (Monopril) Lisinopril (Prinivil, Zestril) Quinapril (Accupril) Ramipril (Altace)	Hypertension, congestive heart failure.	These drugs block or inhibit enzymes necessary to produce angiotensin II, which reduces constriction of the arteries. Thus, the drugs dilate the arteries, improving blood flow and lowering blood pressure. ACE inhibitors also reduce the workload of the heart and improve its performance.	Rash, itching, fever, dizziness, lightheadedness, headaches, low blood pressure.
LIPID-LOWERING DRUGS			
Bile Acid Sequestrants Cholestyramine (Questran, Cholybar) Colestipol (Colestid)	High blood lipids	These drugs lower blood cholesterol by decreasing cholesterol absorption by the intestines, and by increasing the breakdown of LDL cholesterol by the body.	Constipation, bloating, bleeding.

189 •

SOME COMMONLY PRESCRIBED CARDIAC MEDICATIONS (Cont.)

Type of Drug	Prescribed for	How It Works	Potential Side Effects
Bile Acid Sequestrants (Cont.)			
Niacin (Nicobid, Nicolar, Nicotinex)	High blood lipids	These drugs inhibit production of triglycerides and cholesterol in the liver.	Flushing, abnormal liver function tests.
Fibric Acids			
Gemfibrozil (Lopid) Clofibrate (Atromid-s)	High triglycerides	These drugs decrease liver production of triglycerides, increase removal of cholesterol from the liver, and increase production of HDL cholesterol.	Muscle pain (myalgia) and/or inflammation, and rarely possible increases in total cholesterol.
Statins			
Fluvastatin (Lescol) Lovastatin (Mevacor) Pravastatin (Pravachol) Simvastatin (Zocor)	High blood lipids	These drugs inhibit liver enzymes involved in the production of cholesterol and LDL cholesterol.	Few.
Probucol (Lorelco)	High blood lipids	Unknown. Believed to decrease cholesterol production in the liver and increase the breakdown of LDL cholesterol in the bloodstream. Also has antioxidant properties.	Reduces protective HDL cholesterol by 20 to 25 percent. Indigestion, diarrhea.

Type of Drug	Prescribed for	How It Works	Potential Side Effects

DIURETICS

Thiazide Diuretics

Bendroflumethiazide (Naturetin)	Hypertension	These drugs increase the elimination of salt and water by the kidneys, reducing the volume of fluid and the sodium content of the body. Thiazide diuretics also relax the blood vessel walls and dilate the arteries.	Decreased sodium, potassium, and magnesium levels, temporary increases in blood lipids, possible increases in blood sugar, uric acid, increases in blood calcium levels (which possibly help to prevent loss of bone mass in postmenopausal women.)
HydroDIURIL			
Benzthiazide (Aquatag, Exna, Hydrex, Proaqua)			
Chlorothiazide (Diachlor, Diurigen, Diuril)			
Hydrochlorothiazide (HCTZ) (Diuchlor, Esidrix, HydroDIURIL, Mictrin, Oretic, Thiuretic)			
Hydroflumethiazide (Diucardin, Saluron)			
Inapamide (Lozol)			
Methyclothiazide (Aquatensen, Diutensin, Enduron)			
Metolazone (Diulo, Mykrox, Zaroxolyn)			
Polythiazide (Renese)			
Quinethazone (Hydromox)			
Trichlormethiazide (Aquazide, Diurese, Metahydrin, Naqua)			

Potassium/Magnesium-Sparing Diuretics

Amiloride (Midamor)	Hypertension	These drugs prevent reabsorption of sodium and excretion of potassium by the kidneys, thus promoting the loss of sodium and water from the body while retaining potassium.	Increased potassium levels, excessive hair growth.
Spironolactone (Aldactone)			
Triamterene (Dyrenium)			

191 •

Type of Drug	Prescribed for	How It Works	Potential Side Effects
ADRENERGIC INHIBITORS			
Peripheral Adrenergic Antagonists			
Deserpidine (Harmonyl) Guanadrel (Hylorel) Guanethidine (Ismelin) Reserpine (Serpasil, Serpalan) Rescinnamine (Moderil)	Hypertension	These drugs block the actions of the sympathetic nervous system, indirectly dilating the arteries.	Low blood pressure, fatigue, depression, slow pulse, sexual problems.
Central Adrenergic Inhibitors			
Clonidine (Catapres) Guanabenz (Wytensin) Guanfacine (Tenex) Methyldopa (Aldomet)	Hypertension	These drugs decrease the central nervous system's release of norepinephrine, decreasing constriction of blood vessels.	Fatigue, lethargy, rebound hypertension after the drug is stopped, depression, sexual problems.
Alpha Adrenergic Receptor Blocker Drugs			
Doxazosin Mesylate (Cardura) Prazosin (Minipress) Terazocin (Hytrin) Phenoxybenzamine (Dibenzyline) Phentolamine Mesylate (Regitine)	Hypertension	These drugs block the actions of alpha receptors in the sympathetic nervous system, causing the blood vessels to dilate.	Low blood pressure upon sitting or standing.
VASODILATORS			
Hydralazine (Alazine, Apresoline) Minoxidil (Loniten, Minodyl)	Resistant or uncontrolled hypertension	These drugs directly dilate the blood vessels, which lowers blood pressure.	Low blood pressure, water retention, worsening of angina, excessive growth of body hair (Minoxidil).

Coronary Angioplasty

This nonsurgical procedure, known also as *percutaneous transluminal coronary angioplasty* (PTCA), or "balloon" angioplasty, has revolutionized the treatment of coronary artery disease over the last ten years. The procedure, in which a tiny balloon attached to a catheter is used to open clogged coronary arteries, is a less invasive and less expensive alternative to bypass surgery. But it is not for everybody. And although the procedure overall has a 90 percent success rate, it has been documented to be somewhat more risky for women than it is for men.

Who Is a Candidate?

When determining whether or not you are a candidate for PTCA, your doctor will consider your age, the overall functioning of your heart, how long you've had angina, how many of your vessels are narrowed, how severe the narrowing is, and how much calcification (hardening) of the plaque has occurred. Your overall health will be considered, as well.

Although the procedure is most successful when only one coronary artery is narrowed, sometimes multiple PTCAs can be performed when more than one blood vessel is involved.

You *may not* be a good candidate for PTCA if

- you have a plaque that surrounds a curve in the artery or one that is located too far away to be reached by the catheter
- you have severe calcification of a plaque
- you have a plaque in the left main coronary artery
- you have complete blockage of one or more coronary arteries

The Procedure

PTCA is performed in the hospital, under sedation, with a catheter similar to that used for cardiac catheterization (see page 78). After you have received a sedative to relax you, your physician first inserts a catheter into an artery in your arm or leg. With the help of an X-ray camera known as a fluoroscope, the catheter is then guided through the aorta and into the coronary arteries (see Figure 11 on page 194). Once the catheter is in place, a second, smaller catheter equipped with a balloon about the size of a pencil eraser is passed through the first catheter. When the balloon tip reaches the narrowed part of the coronary artery, it is inflated, compressing the plaque and enlarging the diameter of the blood vessel. The balloon is then deflated and the catheters are removed.

FIGURE 11 — Balloon Angioplasty

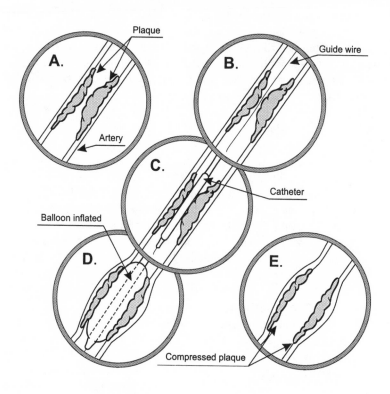

A. Artery obstructed by plaque
B. Guide wire maneuvered through artery using x-ray control
C. Balloon-tipped catheter is laced over guide wire
D. Balloon is inflated resulting in compression of plaque
E. Artery remains open when catheter is removed

You will be carefully observed for several hours after undergoing the procedure. You can usually go home from the hospital two or three days later.

The Risks

Complications associated with PTCA, while relatively rare, are fairly serious. A blood vessel can rupture, a plaque can be dislodged from the artery wall, causing an occlusion of the artery further downstream, or a coronary artery can be torn. All of these complications are potentially life threatening, and some require emergency coronary bypass surgery. For this reason, an emergency heart surgery team is on standby whenever PTCAs are done.

Overall, the rate of complications associated with PTCA is 3 to 5 percent. But several disturbing studies have found the risk of serious complications during the procedure to be somewhat higher for women than for men. It's not clear yet why this is so, but women's smaller body size and the fact that they are older than men when they undergo the procedure, and have more risk factors, such as hypertension and diabetes, all appear to contribute to the higher complication rate. Still, women who successfully come through the period immediately following the procedure seem to fare better than men. The number of women who need repeat PTCA, bypass surgery, or who suffer a heart attack after the procedure, is actually lower than for men.

Is Balloon Angioplasty Right for You?

The main advantages of PTCA are that it relieves angina better than medication alone, and the procedure itself is far less risky, less costly, and less invasive than bypass surgery. PTCA also is associated with a much shorter hospital stay and recovery time than bypass surgery.

Still, because the complication rate associated with the procedure itself is higher in women than men, you should carefully consider this option with the other treatment options available to you. The good news is that new procedures are being developed that may eventually prove to be more effective and less risky for women. These include balloon catheters that are also equipped with miniature lasers, shavers, or cutters.

For now, it appears that women most at risk during PTCA are those age sixty-five and older with multiple risk factors for coronary artery disease. If you are under age sixty-five and are otherwise in good health, your chances of having a successful and uncomplicated PTCA are quite good.

Bypass Surgery

If you have a major blockage (75 percent or more occlusion) of two or all three of the major coronary arteries, or if your left main coronary artery is severely narrowed, you may be a candidate for *coronary artery bypass graft surgery* (CABG). Bypass surgery may be recommended if other medical interventions, including medication or balloon angioplasty, haven't improved your condition.

The operation involves removing a section of blood vessel from another part of the body (either the *saphenous* vein in the leg, or an artery from behind the breastbone, known as the *right* or *left mammary artery*) and using it to bypass the obstructed coronary arteries, thus increasing blood flow to the heart (see Figure 12 on page 197).

Who Is a Candidate?

You may be considered for CAGB if you

- have angina caused by 75 percent or more occlusion of two or all three main coronary arteries
- have narrowing of 75 percent or more of the left main coronary artery
- have no symptoms but have a positive exercise stress test or thallium stress test indicating that all three coronary arteries are almost totally blocked
- have severe narrowing of only one coronary artery but are not a good candidate for PTCA
- have unsuccessfully undergone PTCA

If you have had previous bypass surgeries whose grafts have closed, or if atherosclerosis has developed in previously unaffected areas of the coronary arteries or in the grafts themselves, you may be a candidate for repeat bypass surgery.

The Procedure

CABG is major surgery that is performed in the hospital under general anesthesia. You will probably be admitted to the hospital two or three days before your operation for preoperative tests.

The operation itself may take from three to six hours, depending on how many grafts you must have. (Although there are only three main coronary arteries, it is possible to have four or even five bypasses, rather

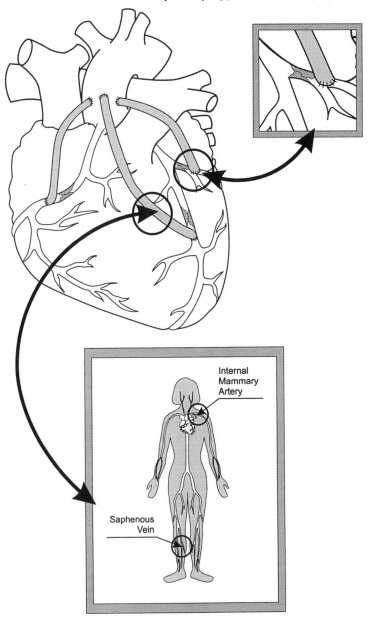

FIGURE 12 — Coronary Artery Bypass Graft Surgery

Internal
Mammary
Artery

Saphenous
Vein

than just three. This is because sometimes the branches off the main arteries are also bypassed.)

During the operation, the surgeon will make an incision through the middle of the chest and through the breastbone, exposing the heart. If a vein is taken from your leg, another incision will be made in your leg. If more than one bypass is needed, it's possible that more than one incision will be made in one or both legs, or in the groin.

Once the heart is exposed, you will be placed on an artificial bypass pump, which pumps blood to the rest of the organs in the body while the heart is cooled to the point that it stops and the bypass grafts are sewn into position. Once the grafts are in place, the heart is warmed or electroshock treatments are used to restart the heart, and the incisions are closed.

After the operation, you will be taken to a recovery room or (more likely) an intensive care unit. Lung and chest tubes may remain in place for up to twenty-four hours to check for internal bleeding. But after the first twenty-four hours, recovery from CABG is fairly swift: By the first postoperative day, you should be totally alert, and able to eat and walk around. If you don't develop any serious complications, you should be out of the hospital within five days.

The Risks
Coronary artery bypass surgery sounds risky (after all, the heart is stopped while the grafts are sewn in place) and, like any operation, some risk is involved. The most serious risk is dying during surgery. For a healthy patient with no other complicating factors, such risk is quite low—only 1 to 2 percent. Unfortunately, numerous studies have consistently found that the risk of dying during surgery is somewhat higher for women than it is for men. When the nine major studies investigating the risks of CABG to women are combined, the relative risk is more than twice as high as that for men.

Although initially these statistics sound alarming, they must be put into perspective. Overall, while men have about a 2 percent mortality rate associated with the operation, women have a 5 percent mortality rate. *But this still means that 95 percent of women will survive the operation.*

No one is sure yet why the mortality rate for women undergoing bypass surgery is higher than it is for men. Some studies have suggested that the mortality rate has decreased over time, as surgical techniques have improved, and that women are no longer at a greater risk than men. Others have found the difference between men and women to be primarily a result of differences in the size of the coronary arteries. The National Institutes of Health's CASS study, for example, found that shorter patients, whether male or female, had higher mortality rates than taller patients. The higher mortality rate also may be due to the fact that women who undergo bypass surgery generally are older and sicker than men having the operation.

Another drawback to the surgery is that it doesn't bring as much relief from angina for women as it does for men.

In spite of the somewhat greater risk to women at the time of surgery and the fact that it is less successful in easing angina in women, the long-term outlook for women who successfully undergo the procedure is good. In fact, there is not much difference in five-and ten-year survival rates between men and women who have had bypass surgery. On average, five-year survival ranges from 87 to 91 percent in women, compared with 90 to 94 percent in men. As mentioned earlier, at least one study has found that women who use postmenopausal estrogens after CABG have better five- and ten-year survival rates than those who don't use estrogen.

Should You Have Bypass Surgery?

If your physician recommends bypass surgery, make sure you understand why bypass surgery is preferable to angioplasty, a much less invasive procedure. You should also ask what the surgery will accomplish, what medications you might need to take after bypass surgery, how long the benefits of surgery are expected to last, and what kind of recovery time you can expect.

If you have any doubts about your doctor's recommendation, by all means get a second, and possibly a third, opinion. In fact, many insurance companies require a second opinion for such procedures as angioplasty and bypass surgery.

What About Lifestyle Changes?

Reducing your risk of a heart attack with lifestyle changes alone is, of course, preferable to medication and surgery simply because there are virtually no dangerous side effects associated with changing your eating and exercise habits (except, perhaps, sustaining an exercise-related injury, which can easily be prevented), so safety isn't a serious issue, as it is with, say, bypass surgery.

What about effectiveness? There's some evidence that lifestyle changes can be quite effective in reversing the development of plaques and restoring blood flow to the heart, especially in women. One of the first formal studies to suggest that artery-narrowing plaques can be shrunk involved a combination of diet and drugs. The study, published in 1990, involved forty-one women and thirty-one men with the genetic disorder *familial hypercholesterolemia*, which causes abnormally high cholesterol levels. All of the volunteers had a baseline coronary angiogram indicating significant narrowing of the coronary arteries. Then the men and women were divided into two groups: the control group received diet counseling along with the cholesterol-lowering drug colestipol. The treatment group received diet counseling and a combination of cholesterol-lowering drugs.

At the end of the study, the women in the treatment group experienced a significant regression of coronary lesions, whereas those in the control group had a progressive increase in the size of their lesions. And the regression of plaques in the treated women was much greater than that in the treated men.

Dean Ornish, M.D., and his colleagues at the University of California, demonstrated that, even without drugs, an extremely low-fat diet combined with regular moderate exercise and stress-reducing techniques, could in fact *reverse* narrowing of artery-clogging plaques within a year. Interestingly, the one woman in the experimental group experienced the greatest degree of plaque regression. But even women in the comparison group, who followed the American Heart Association's Step I diet (30 percent fat) and who were counseled on reducing other risk factors, had some regression of their plaques as well. Preliminary results of follow-up studies have confirmed these early findings.

As encouraging as these studies are, the results should still be considered preliminary. Should you decide to follow a program of lifestyle intervention, you should keep in mind that making even minor lifestyle changes can be a challenge. The people in these studies made fairly drastic lifestyle changes, and they had plenty of professional support and encouragement to help them stick with the rigorous diet, exercise, and stress-management regimen associated with regression of plaques in the coronary arteries. You, too, will need a good dose of self-determination, along with heaping helpings of support from your family, friends, physician, and other members of your treatment team.

Even if you *don't* rely on dramatic lifestyle changes alone as a treatment option, most of the medical treatments for coronary artery disease are more effective when combined with such risk-reducing strategies as a low-fat diet, exercise, and stress management. In fact, some physicians refuse to offer bypass surgery to patients who won't quit smoking or make other lifestyle changes to lower their risk. And so far, the research strongly suggests that making lifestyle changes can have a big payoff: You may require less medication, and will enjoy the benefits of invasive procedures such as angioplasty and bypass surgery for much longer than if you continue to eat a high-fat diet, lead a sedentary lifestyle, and continue smoking. At the very least, you'll feel better. And who knows—you may even be able to reverse some of the damage that has already been done to your arteries.

CHAPTER 12

If You Have a Heart Attack

HAVING A HEART ATTACK is one of the most serious consequences of coronary artery disease. Even if you are following the guidelines in this book for preventing heart trouble, it is a good idea to prepare yourself for dealing with a heart attack—just in case. This is especially true if you have any of the major risk factors for heart disease or if you have already been diagnosed with coronary artery disease.

The good news is that treatment advances in the last ten to fifteen years have vastly improved the outlook for people who suffer a heart attack: *Of the estimated 1.5 million Americans who will have a heart attack this year, roughly two-thirds will survive.* And many survivors continue to lead full, productive lives. You can too.

In this chapter, you'll learn how to determine whether you are having a heart attack, what to do about it, and what you can expect in terms of treatment and recovery from the ordeal.

Am I Having a Heart Attack?

If you happen to have a heart attack, you can dramatically increase your odds of surviving the ordeal by knowing the warning signs and seeking prompt medical treatment. *Denying the problem or ignoring the symptoms can cost you your life.*

Unfortunately, as Susan's story illustrates, it isn't always easy to tell when you are having a heart attack. Susan, a fifty-three-year-old house-mother of a fraternity house on the University of Florida campus, recalls her symptoms.

Case Report: Susan

On the morning of my heart attack, I woke up feeling fine. But by 9:00 or 9:30 A.M., I started to notice a pressure in my chest. When I returned from the grocery store that morning, I set the grocery bags down in the kitchen and told the cook, "I don't feel too well. I don't know what's going on here." I thought I might have indigestion so I took an antacid. At about 11:00 A.M., as I was talking with the accountant, my arms started to ache. That's when I knew something serious was going on.

After the accountant left, I called Dr. Notelovitz's clinic. The receptionist was alert enough to get one of the doctors instead of having a nurse call me back. I explained to the doctor that I felt a pressure in my chest and my arms felt achy, and that I had taken an antacid thinking that it was indigestion. She looked at my chart and said, "Susan, you're not a candidate for heart attack." She recommended that I come to the clinic just the same.

When I got there, I guess I didn't look too good. The nurse called me back to an examination room and did an ECG. While the test was in progress, I started breaking out in a sweat and feeling nauseous. That's when they said, "Susan, you're having a heart attack." They gave me nitroglycerine and called an ambulance to take me to the hospital.

Chest Pain: What to Look for, What to Do

Although not all chest pain is caused by a heart attack, chest pain or discomfort should not be ignored. In the event that your chest pain *is* caused by a heart attack, the more quickly you receive medical treatment, the more likely you will be to survive the episode with minimal damage to your heart. But how can you tell the difference between an episode of chest pain that requires immediate medical attention and one that can wait a day or two (or longer) before being evaluated by a physician?

Generally speaking, the chest pain caused by a heart attack or angina is more of a discomfort or ache rather than a sharp pain. Some terms commonly used by heart patients to describe the pain are "pressure," "heaviness," "squeezing," and "tightness." Some patients describe a "burning sensation" that feels like indigestion. Stabbing chest pain usually *is not* associated with a heart attack or angina.

The pain of a heart attack doesn't necessarily arise from the left side of the chest, either. The discomfort can occur anywhere in the chest. Typically, it manifests as a deep central discomfort below the breastbone. Sometimes the pain spreads to the shoulder, arms, upper back,neck, or jaw. Conversely, if you can pinpoint the exact location of the pain and the main source of the pain covers an area no larger than the size of a coin, chances are good that it is not caused by a heart attack.

How long the pain lasts can also provide clues as to the cause. Fleeting pains that last just a few seconds usually do not signal a heart attack or angina. A heart attack is associated with chest discomfort lasting fifteen minutes or more. Anginal symptoms tend to come and go, lasting anywhere from two to five minutes, and are often preceded by an increase in physical activity, emotional stress, or exposure to cold weather.

What should you do if you develop chest pain? If you are over age thirty-five and the pain persists for more than a few minutes, you should seek immediate medical attention. The American Heart Association advises you to call 911 or the local emergency service number if you have any of the following symptoms:

- An uncomfortable pressure, fullness, squeezing, or pain in the center of the chest that does not go away in a few minutes
- Pain spreading to the shoulders, neck, or arms
- Chest discomfort accompanied by lightheadedness and palpitations, fainting, sweating, nausea, or shortness of breath

If you already have angina and the pain persists after taking nitroglycerine or aspirin, you should go directly to the hospital emergency room or call 911. *Do not delay.* (If you are not taken to the hospital by ambulance, *do not* take public transportation or drive yourself; have a family member or friend drive you.)

Even if you have other types of chest pain, you should at least call your doctor if the episodes persist.

What Happens If You Have a Heart Attack

When you are having a heart attack, every minute counts. Ideally, you should seek emergency medical help within fifteen minutes of the onset of chest pain. If you can get to the hospital within four hours of the onset of your symptoms—and at the very latest, six hours—emergency medical personnel can begin therapy with drugs that break up the blood clot that likely caused the heart attack, therefore minimizing the damage to your heart.

Your initial evaluation in the emergency room will include a check of your vital signs, including your heart rate and rhythm with an ECG. You will have blood tests to check for elevated levels of certain enzymes that signify you are having a heart attack. An IV infusion will be started to provide speedy access for drug therapies that may be needed. You will also receive pain medication to help you feel more comfortable.

Once you have been diagnosed as having a heart attack, emergency room doctors will quickly work to return the heart to a normal rhythm and to restore blood flow to the heart muscle.

Treating Arrhythmias

The first priority will be to treat arrhythmias. This is critical, since proper blood flow is dependent on a regular heart rhythm. If you are awake and alert, lidocaine will be administered through your IV to help return your heart to a normal rhythm. If you are unconscious, it may be necessary for medical personnel to perform cardiopulmonary resuscitation (CPR) or to apply electroshock treatments to the heart with a defibrillator.

Thrombolytic Therapy

After the heartbeat is restored to a normal rhythm, the underlying cause of heart attack itself can be treated. This is done with the help of "clot-busting" drugs that have revolutionized the treatment of heart attacks over the past fifteen years. These drugs include *streptokinase* (KabiKinase, Streptase), *urokinase* (Abbokinase, Win-Kinase), *tissue-plasminogen activator (tPA)* (Activase), and *anistreplase* (Eminase). The drugs work by dissolving the tough fibrin strands that hold a blood clot together, which in turn breaks up the clot.

Thrombolytic drugs have been found to work as well in women as in men in breaking up clots, and thrombolytic therapy has been found to reduce mortality rates in both men and women dramatically. But several major studies have found that the reduction in mortality rates among women receiving these drugs—31 percent in one study—is still considerably lower than among men, whose mortality was reduced by 45 percent in the same study.

There are many possible reasons for the gender disparity in the ability of clot busting drugs to save lives. Some scientists speculate that the older age of women at the time of a heart attack contributes to their relatively lower reduction in mortality, although not all studies support this theory. Others point to studies showing that women are more vulnerable than men to complications related to the use of these drugs, specifically bleeding. In one study involving the use of tPA, 5.9 percent of women versus 3.8 percent of men developed major bleeding problems. The differences in complication rates are thought to be partly related to the smaller body size of women who, pound for pound, receive more of the drug than men given the same dose.

Another, more serious problem women face is whether or not they will even receive these life-saving drugs for the treatment of a heart attack. In one study, only 55 percent of eligible women received tPA, compared with 78 percent of eligible men of the same age. The study authors gave no explanation for the gender differences in the use of tPA.

Of course, not everyone is a candidate for thrombolytic therapy. If you have an active peptic ulcer or known gastrointestinal bleeding, if you have had a hemorrhagic stroke, or if you have severe anemia, you should not get these drugs. If you have had previous injections of streptokinase or urokinase, you are more likely to develop an allergic reaction after receiving repeated injections. Instead, you may have to use the more expensive thrombolytic agent, tPA. Because it is genetically engineered from a human protein, tPA is not associated with allergic reactions.

Because there is evidence that women are less likely to receive thrombolytic therapy than men, you should ask your doctor—in advance—whether there is a good reason why you *should not* receive these drugs in the event you have a heart attack.

Angioplasty and Bypass Surgery

Using angioplasty and coronary bypass surgery as emergency treatment to restore blood flow to the heart is controversial because the heart is extremely vulnerable right after a heart attack, and the procedures themselves carry the risk of triggering another heart attack. Only in the most unusual cases are the procedures warranted. Most physicians prefer to wait until after you have recovered from your heart attack to open clogged coronary arteries with angioplasty, or bypass them altogether with coronary bypass surgery. (For more on these procedures, see Chapter 11.)

Other Drugs

After you've had a heart attack, you may receive additional medications to aid in your recovery.

Antiarrhythmic drugs. The heart is particularly prone to developing irregular rhythms immediately after a heart attack. These drugs are commonly given to reduce the occurrence of abnormal heart rhythms.

Beta-blockers. These drugs may be given to slow your heart rate, reduce the likelihood of arrhythmias, and increase blood flow to the heart after a heart attack. If you have high blood pressure, beta-blockers will also help to lower it. Beta-blockers have been associated with improved survival of both men and women who take them after a heart attack.

ACE Inhibitors. Recent studies (most of which have involved men) have shown that these drugs are associated with increased survival when given after a heart attack. Patients who appear to benefit most are those with left ventricular hypertrophy and systolic blood pressure (the top number of a blood pressure reading) over 100 mm/Hg.

Aspirin or other antiplatelet agents. Aspirin is the most commonly used antiplatelet drug. It is given after a heart attack to prevent blood clots from forming in the arteries.

Anticoagulants. Heparin and warfarin are often given along with aspirin to help prevent the formation of new blood clots in heart attack patients.

Nitroglycerine. Nitrates dilate the coronary arteries, increasing blood flow to the heart and relieving the pain of angina.

Narcotics. These may be given to help relieve the pain and the anxiety that typically accompany a heart attack.

Your Physical Recovery

After your initial treatment in the emergency room, you will be moved to a coronary care unit (CCU), where you will be constantly monitored to minimize any further damage to your heart.

When your condition has stabilized, you will be moved to an intermediate care unit, where you will continue to be monitored, and where your rehabilitation begins. You will probably be encouraged to get out of bed and walk around within a few days. And if there are no complications, you can expect to return home within a week.

Before you leave the hospital, you will probably undergo an exercise stress test to determine whether or not you will develop angina. You will also be given advice on nutrition, exercise, and other risk-reducing strategies that can help you prevent a second heart attack.

You will be advised to increase your level of activity gradually. Generally speaking you can expect to progress from light housework within a week or two of your discharge from the hospital, to more vigorous activities, including sexual intercourse, within three or four weeks—provided you don't have any shortness of breath or pain.

It takes about three months to fully recover from a heart attack. After about six weeks, you can expect to take a more vigorous exercise stress test to determine whether or not you would benefit from angioplasty or coronary bypass surgery.

Your Emotional Recovery

While your physical recovery from a heart attack takes just a few months, your emotional recovery may take much longer. You've just survived a life-threatening experience, one that has undoubtedly left you feeling vulnerable, deeply concerned about your health, and terrified that you might have another heart attack.

The fear of having another heart attack can be crippling. Some women are afraid to leave the house for even brief periods of time after having a heart attack. Remember, fear can be a powerful motivator. If fear of having another heart attack begins to paralyze you, try to redirect your energies toward making lifestyle changes that will aid in your recovery.

Preventing a Second Heart Attack

Many of the same recommendations for preventing coronary artery disease are also essential for the treatment of existing heart disease and for rehabilitation after a heart attack. Your plan for preventing a second heart attack should include a low-fat, low-cholesterol diet similar to the one outlined in Chapter 6, regular moderate exercise (see page 126 for specific guidelines for people with existing heart disease), plans to quit smoking and to control stress, and aggressive treatment of hypertension and diabetes. You may also have to continue taking beta-blockers, aspirin, or other cardiac medications prescribed by your doctor.

After you've had a heart attack, your life may never be the same as it was before. To prevent another heart attack from happening, you'll need to make changes in your lifestyle, and you may have to take medication for the rest of your life. This is not to say that you must resign yourself to a life of deprivation, drugs, and dependency. Many people who've had a heart attack go on to lead full, productive, and very long lives.

Crisis is the Chinese word for danger—and opportunity. Try to view this experience as a unique opportunity to review your priorities and commitments in life, and to renew your commitment to take care of yourself and to do the things that mean the most to you. Thus, you may find that your heart attack is a catalyst for making the rest of your life better than ever.

PART III

Other Forms of Cardiovascular Disease

CHAPTER 13

Hypertension

IF THERE'S ONE type of heart disease that's an equal-opportunity killer, it's hypertension, or high blood pressure. Half of the estimated fifty million Americans with hypertension are women. And while we're not sure why, after menopause your chances of having high blood pressure are greater than a man's.

Fortunately, your risk of having a heart attack or stroke can be significantly reduced by keeping your blood pressure in check.

What Is Hypertension?

In simplest terms, hypertension is excessive force of blood on the artery walls as it is pumped from the heart. Normally, the arteries help maintain a steady supply of blood from your head to your toes by dilating and contracting as needed so that, for instance, when you stand up, the blood supply to your brain isn't compromised as the forces of gravity work to pull the blood down toward your feet.

When you have high blood pressure, the arteries remain constricted. As a result, the heart and arteries must strain to pump blood through the body.

Most people with elevated blood pressure have what's known as *essential* or *primary* hypertension, which has no known cause. However, about 5 percent of people with high blood pressure have *secondary hypertension*— high blood pressure that is a symptom of an underlying medical problem that, when treated, causes blood pressure to return to normal. If your blood pressure doesn't fall after drug therapy, or if your blood pressure suddenly worsens, your physician may look for an underlying cause.

Another type of hypertension that is receiving increasing attention is *isolated systolic hypertension*, which occurs when systolic blood pressure is elevated but diastolic pressure is not. Women over age fifty are more likely to have isolated systolic hypertension than men.

Some women develop hypertension during pregnancy, a condition known by many terms, including pregnancy-induced hypertension, pre-eclampsia, eclampsia, or toxemia.

A Silent Killer

Although high blood pressure is generally symptomless, the dangers of untreated hypertension are numerous and potentially deadly. Over time, the arteries may become scarred, hardened, and less elastic, making them unable to carry adequate amounts of blood to the body's organs. The heart, brain, and kidneys are most vulnerable. People with hypertension *and* high cholesterol levels are more likely to develop artery-narrowing plaques, a condition known as *atherosclerosis*. Among these people, there's a greater risk that a blood clot circulating in the bloodstream will get lodged in arteries narrowed by atherosclerosis and cut off the blood supply to surrounding tissues, triggering a life-threatening heart attack or stroke. In fact, hypertension is the most important risk factor for stroke, and one of the major risk factors for coronary heart disease.

High blood pressure can also cause the heart to enlarge and become less efficient, a condition known as *left ventricular hypertrophy*. This condition can, over time, weaken the heart and lead to heart failure.

Even "Mild" Hypertension Is Dangerous

Until recently, the serious consequences of hypertension were believed to be most threatening to people with moderate to severe hypertension. However, new studies have demonstrated that even people with mildly elevated blood pressure—the kind most affected people have—are at a substantially greater risk for premature death from a heart attack or stroke and a wide variety of complications associated with hypertension, including organ damage. An estimated 60 percent of deaths attributed to hypertension-induced coronary artery disease in the U.S. occur in people with so-called mild hypertension.

Who Is at Risk for Hypertension?

Some women are more likely to develop hypertension than others. Do you have any of the following risk factors?

Your Age
Your risk of developing hypertension increases as you grow older. Generally speaking, the older you get, the more likely you are to develop high blood pressure.

Your Ethnic Background
No one is sure why, but, at any given age, more black women have hypertension than white women. Black women ages sixty-five and older are especially at risk.

A Family History of Hypertension
If your parents have high blood pressure, you are more likely to develop it yourself.

"High Normal" Blood Pressure
According to the Joint National Committee on the Detection, Evaluation and Treatment of High Blood Pressure, if your blood pressure is above normal (over 130/85), but not high enough to be diagnosed as hypertension, you should consider yourself at risk of developing high blood pressure at some point in the future, and should take appropriate measures to prevent this from happening. Your risk of developing hypertension is also increased if you experience a progressive increase within the range of "normal" blood pressure.

Your Weight
Overweight women (more than 30 percent over their ideal weight) are two to three times more likely to develop high blood pressure than women of normal weight.

A High-Sodium Diet
From one-third to one-half of all people with hypertension are "salt-sensitive"; that is, their blood pressure rises when on a high-sodium diet and falls on a low-sodium diet.

Preliminary research suggests that a low intake of calcium, potassium, or magnesium may also be associated with an increased risk.

A History of Pregnancy-Induced Hypertension
If you developed high blood pressure during a past pregnancy, you are at a greater risk of developing hypertension later in life.

Heavy Use of Alcohol
You've probably heard that alcohol helps protect against cardiovascular disease. This is not necessarily so when it comes to hypertension. Consuming three or more drinks per day is associated with an *increased* incidence of hypertension. One study found that women who consumed more than three drinks per day increased their risk of developing hypertension by 90 percent.

Diabetes
For reasons that are not entirely understood, people with diabetes are at greater risk of developing high blood pressure. A growing body of evidence has now demonstrated that the high insulin levels characteristic of non-insulin-dependent diabetes play a key role in the development of hypertension.

Use of Oral Contraceptives
A small number of women—less than 5 percent—will develop high blood pressure while using oral contraceptives. Most at risk are women who are already at risk of developing hypertension: African-American women, those who are overweight and/or over age forty, those who have had hypertension during pregnancy, those who have a family history of hypertension, or women with mild kidney disease.

If you develop high blood pressure while taking oral contraceptives, your physician will probably advise you to stop taking them. Blood pressure usually returns to normal within a few months after you stop taking the Pill.

Stress
Many people think of high blood pressure as a "stress" disease, caused by overworking and other modern-day pressures. Some studies *have* suggested that chronic stress can lead to permanent increases in heart rate and blood pressure. For instance, male air traffic controllers, who hold high-pressure jobs, have two to four times the rate of hypertension, compared to men of similar age in other occupations. No studies to date have involved women.

That's not to say that stress *causes* hypertension. As we mentioned earlier, we don't know yet what causes high blood pressure. But stress can contribute to the problem.

What about menopause? Most studies, including our own, have found that menopause has no significant effect on blood pressure. Rather, the gradual rise in blood pressure as you grow older appears to be a part of the normal aging process.

Making a Diagnosis

Many people have high blood pressure for years without knowing it. This is why it is paramount to have your blood pressure checked periodically. Most physicians, including gynecologists, now regularly check your blood pressure every time you visit.

Remember, a blood pressure reading is written as a fraction consisting of two numbers. The top number, or *systolic pressure*, represents blood pressure while the heart is beating. The bottom number, *diastolic pressure*, represents blood pressure while the heart is at rest. A reading of 120/80 is considered normal for most people.

In light of recent research demonstrating that even mildly elevated blood pressure can lead to organ damage and an increased risk of heart attack or stroke, the Joint National Committee on the Detection, Evaluation, and Treatment of High Blood Pressure has proposed a new classification system for high blood pressure that de-emphasizes the use of such terms as "mild" and "moderate" hypertension. The new system uses stages to classify high blood pressure (see "Blood Pressure Classification for Adults 18 and Older," on page 216). The report's authors point out that while people with higher blood pressure are at a greater risk, "*all* stages of hypertension are associated with increased risk of cardiovascular and kidney disease."

The report also emphasizes the importance of elevated *systolic* pressure as a gauge in diagnosing and treating patients. In the past, physicians relied mainly on diastolic pressure to determine who should be treated, and how. But studies involving elderly women and men demonstrated that aggressive treatment of systolic hypertension significantly reduced the incidence of stroke and heart problems. So if your systolic pressure is elevated even when your diastolic pressure is within the normal range, a condition known as *isolated systolic hypertension*, your doctor will recommend that you be treated.

If your doctor finds that your blood pressure is elevated during a routine office visit, it doesn't necessarily mean you have high blood pressure. Your

BLOOD PRESSURE CLASSIFICATION FOR ADULTS 18 AND OLDER

CATEGORY	SYSTOLIC mm/Hg	DIASTOLIC mm/Hg
Normal	less than 130	less than 85
High normal	130–139	85–89
Hypertension		
Stage I (mild)	140–159	90–99
Stage II (moderate)	160–179	100–109
Stage III (severe)	180–209	110–119
Stage IV (very severe)	210 or greater	120 or greater

blood pressure varies widely over time, depending on many variables. Blood pressure often rises when you are nervous or excited, for example, but normally it goes down again almost immediately. In fact, some 15 percent of people with Stage I hypertension may actually have what's called "white-coat hypertension," in which their blood pressure is elevated only at the doctor's office. (Note: Because caffeine and nicotine can temporarily raise your blood pressure, be sure to avoid cigarettes and caffeine-containing beverages just before having your blood pressure checked.) If your blood pressure is above 140/90, your physician will want to measure it again on at least two subsequent visits before making a diagnosis of hypertension.

A Lifestyle for Lowering Blood Pressure

If you have Stage I hypertension or mild isolated systolic hypertension and no other risk factors for cardiovascular disease, your physician may first recommend that you try certain lifestyle changes to help lower it. If you have "high normal" blood pressure, you should also follow the recommendations here as a preventive measure.

Lifestyle modifications can be highly effective at lowering blood pressure ... but only if you are motivated to stick with them. Here are some of the ways you can work to reduce your blood pressure without medication.

Lose Weight

If you weigh more than 10 percent over your ideal body weight (ask your doctor, or check the height and weight tables on page 286), losing weight is perhaps *the* most effective way to lower blood pressure without medication. According to a study in the *Archives of Internal Medicine*, if you have Stage 1 hypertension, you don't need to lose much weight—on average about seven pounds—to return blood pressure to normal. What's more, most of the people in that study who initially lost weight maintained normal blood pressure even after gaining some or all of the weight back, report researchers at the University of Texas School of Public Health. Most experts caution, however, that weight loss works only if you keep most of the weight off, and regaining weight is a common problem.

A sensible, low-fat diet, combined with regular, moderate exercise is most effective. For long-term success, support groups such as Weight Watchers, Overeaters Anonymous, and Taking Off Pounds Sensibly may be of help.

Exercise

Regular, moderate exercise has been shown to be *as effective as medication* for lowering mildly to moderately elevated blood pressure. According to the Joint National Committee, "physical activity need not be complicated or expensive; for most sedentary people, such moderate activity as thirty to forty-five minutes of brisk walking three to five times per week will be beneficial." Exercise lowers blood pressure by helping the heart to work more efficiently. It also works indirectly by helping overweight people lose weight.

Even if you take drugs to lower your blood pressure, you can often reduce the amount you take by exercising regularly. At her first visit to our clinic, fifty-seven-year-old Martha Watson's blood pressure was 160/100. We prescribed a mild diuretic and, after administering an exercise stress test, gave her the green light to begin a regular program of exercise, including a brisk twenty- to thirty-minute walk three times per week. Several months later, Martha's blood pressure had decreased to 118/78, as a result of exercise and, to a lesser extent, her medication. We therefore were able to reduce her medication significantly.

If you have high blood pressure and want to begin an exercise program, you should do so *only* after you've had a complete medical evaluation by your physician, and only under your doctor's supervision. (See Chapter 7 for instructions on beginning an exercise program.)

Cut Back on Alcohol

Having as few as three drinks per day can not only raise blood pressure but also make you resistant to antihypertensive therapy. If you currently have three or more drinks per day, reducing your alcohol consumption can significantly lower your blood pressure. (If you are not a heavy drinker to begin with and you stop drinking altogether, you may not see much change in your blood pressure.) *All* women with hypertension, as well as those with high-normal blood pressure, should limit their alcohol consumption to two drinks per day or fewer (one drink equals one ounce of hard liquor, four ounces of wine, or twelve ounces of beer).

Shake the Salt Habit

This is one of the most common and, according to some experts, most effective ways to lower blood pressure. It is also one of the most controversial.

A low-sodium diet lowers systolic blood pressure by a modest five to six points. While this may not seem like much, it may be all that is needed to return mildly elevated hypertension to normal. The problem: Sodium restriction is not effective for everyone. Remember, only one-third to one-half of all people with hypertension are sodium sensitive. The recommendation may not work for the other one-half to two-thirds of hypertensive patients who try it. Those most responsive to sodium restriction include women of African-American ancestry, older women, and those with established hypertension.

Another pitfall is that many people don't cut down sufficiently on sodium for this recommendation to work. Reducing sodium intake to 2300 milligrams per day (the amount in a little more than a teaspoon of salt) is the current recommendation. But some studies suggest that to lower blood pressure, a more drastic reduction may be necessary, and this can be difficult to do.

In spite of the controversy over the effectiveness of sodium restriction, the Joint National Committee, the American Heart Association, and the National Heart, Lung and Blood Institute still recommend a low-sodium diet for *all* people with hypertension. Our advice: try reducing your sodium intake for six months. If sodium restriction works, you may have saved yourself a bundle of money by avoiding antihypertensive medication. If you *don't* see any results, don't be too discouraged. You may be one of the hypertensive people who doesn't respond to this recommendation. (For tips on reducing the sodium in your diet, see page 98.)

Keep Up Your Calcium Intake

Calcium does more than build strong teeth and bones. Several population studies have associated a low calcium intake with high blood pressure. Moreover, calcium supplements totaling 1,500 milligrams per day have been shown to lower blood pressure in men.

Although more evidence is needed before we can start prescribing calcium supplements to help control blood pressure, it can't hurt to make sure you're getting plenty of calcium in your diet, especially since calcium has been shown to help prevent osteoporosis, and may even help prevent colon cancer. Women generally *don't* get enough calcium in their diets. (See Chapter 6 for ways to increase the calcium content of your diet.)

Increase Your Intake of Potassium

A low-potassium diet has been associated with high blood pressure. Conversely, potassium supplements have been associated with small reductions in blood pressure. Moreover, if you take antihypertensive drugs, you may find that you need less medication when you take potassium supplements.

To increase your potassium intake, eat plenty of fresh fruits and vegetables. Orange juice, bananas, and potato skins are particularly high in potassium. A single banana contains 451 milligrams of potassium. An eight-ounce glass of orange juice contains 495 milligrams.

Control Stress

Although it is still not certain what role stress plays in the development of hypertension, relaxation techniques such as deep breathing, progressive muscular relaxation, yoga, meditation, and biofeedback can help undo the effects of stress on your body. Relaxation techniques have been found to reduce blood pressure by several points when used in the treatment of hypertension—the higher the blood pressure to begin with, the greater the drop that occurs.

More long-term studies are needed before relaxation therapy can be recommended for the treatment of hypertension. But if you have mild hypertension, you may want to try some of these techniques in conjunction with other non-drug therapies. They can't hurt, and they just might help. (To get started, see "A Simple Way to Relieve Stress," on page 143.)

The Joint National Committee on the Detection, Evaluation and Treatment of Hypertension recommends that you try these lifestyle modifications for six months. There are obvious advantages to doing so, one of which is that they can potentially save you a considerable amount of money (the cost of antihypertensive drugs). You also will be spared the potential side effects of antihypertensive medications. If these measures fail to lower your blood pressure within six months, however, your physician probably won't hesitate to prescribe medication, given what we now know about the health risks of even "mild" hypertension.

Even if you eventually begin taking medication to lower your blood pressure, you should continue to practice these sensible, health-promoting lifestyle modifications anyway, since they can significantly reduce the amount of medication you need, and can lower your overall risk of suffering a heart attack or stroke.

Common Antihypertensive Medications

If your diastolic blood pressure is higher than 95, your systolic pressure is higher than 140 (even if diastolic pressure is not elevated), if you have mildly elevated blood pressure along with other risk factors for coronary artery disease, if you have high blood pressure along with left ventricular hypertrophy, or if lifestyle measures fail to lower even mildly elevated blood pressure, your physician may recommend one of several types of antihypertensive drugs to help bring your blood pressure down. (See "Some Commonly Prescribed Cardiac Medications," on page 186). When used properly, today's blood pressure medications adequately control blood pressure 80 to 90 percent of the time. However, as with any drug therapy, there is the potential for side effects. Your physician will try to bring your blood pressure under control with the minimum dose of drugs and the fewest side effects.

Thiazide Diuretics
These are the most commonly prescribed medications, and the ones physicians often turn to first. These drugs work on the kidneys and rid the body of sodium. Another advantage for women is that thiazide diuretics encourage the reabsorption of calcium by the kidneys, which reduces the risk of hip fractures. Diuretics are cheap, easy to take, and highly effective. However, they may cause fatigue, electrolyte imbalances, and sexual problems (particularly in men).

Beta-Blockers
These drugs slow the heart rate and decrease the contracting power of the heart muscle. They are commonly prescribed for people with symptoms of

coronary artery disease (such as angina pectoris, or chest pain), or people who've had a heart attack. Side effects include fatigue and sexual problems. Some beta-blockers may reduce protective HDL cholesterol.

Angiotensin-Converting Enzyme Inhibitors

Known as ACE inhibitors, these drugs may also be prescribed to help control blood pressure. ACE inhibitors are potent dilators of the arteries and veins, and, in some instances, blood pressure can be markedly lowered with small doses of these drugs. However, people who take ACE inhibitors sometimes develop a rash, a cough, or high potassium levels in their blood.

Calcium Channel Blockers

These drugs, also known as calcium antagonists, dilate the arteries by blocking the entry of calcium into the smooth muscle tissue of the heart and blood vessels. The most bothersome side effects of this drug are headache, water retention (edema), and constipation.

Adrenergic Inhibitors

These drugs help control blood pressure by either stimulating or blocking the activity of the nervous system, either in the brain, elsewhere in the body, or in both places. (Beta-blockers, discussed earlier, fall into this category of drugs.) These drugs are typically prescribed for people with more advanced hypertension. Side effects include low blood pressure, slow pulse, depression, fatigue, and sexual problems, particularly in men.

Vasodilators

These drugs lower blood pressure by dilating the blood vessels, and are usually given to patients in whom other drugs have failed. Because vasodilators may increase the heart rate, they often must be given along with medication to counter this effect.

Estrogen

Although postmenopausal estrogen preparations are not used for the treatment of high blood pressure, these drugs have been found to lower blood pressure in postmenopausal women. In one study of ours, women who took oral estrogens alone experienced nearly a 4 percent decline in systolic blood pressure. (The estrogen patch also lowered blood pressure, but by only 1.5 percent.) The combination of estrogen and exercise really packed a punch: These women experienced a 6 percent decline in blood pressure.

While it is now considered safe for women with hypertension to take estrogen to help ease menopausal symptoms and protect their bones, more research needs to be conducted before estrogen is *routinely* prescribed to help lower blood pressure. But if you have hypertension, you can safely take estrogen without having to worry that it will increase your blood pressure.

Other Benefits of Antihypertensive Medications

In addition to lowering your blood pressure effectively, beta-blockers, ACE inhibitors, and another class of drugs occasionally used to treat hypertension, known as *central alpha agonists*, may also reduce the likelihood of *left ventricular hypertrophy*, a condition in which the heart wall thickens and that can lead to congestive heart failure. The only antihypertensive drugs that *don't* have this protective effect are diuretics. So if your physician prescribes diuretics, he or she may also recommend that you use them in combination with other antihypertensive medications that do help prevent left ventricular hypertrophy.

You may have to visit your doctor as often as once a week when you first start taking blood pressure medication to ensure that the drug is working properly and that you're not suffering any adverse side effects. If you have mild hypertension that has been kept in check with drug therapy for at least a year, your physician may gradually reduce the amount of medication you take, particularly if you also have been using nondrug methods (diet, exercise, weight loss) to help control your blood pressure. However, regular medical checkups are a must, since blood pressure can rise again to hypertensive levels, even after years without therapy.

When Your Blood Pressure Is Too Low

Can your blood pressure be *too low*? Some women, particularly those over age sixty-five, do have a problem with *orthostatic* or *postural hypotension*, a sudden drop in blood pressure when they stand up too quickly or get out of bed in the morning. What happens when you stand or sit up from a lying position is that gravity pulls the blood to your extremities and your brain is temporarily left without an adequate blood supply. The problem may be compounded in older women by the decline in cerebral blood flow that naturally occurs with age, by illness, and by certain medications (see page 224).

Although orthostatic hypotension in itself isn't life threatening, it may produce dizziness, which could cause you to lose your balance and lead to a fall. (Accidents, especially falls, are a leading cause of death among women ages sixty-five and over.)

If you regularly get dizzy when you sit or stand up suddenly, are over age sixty-five, or have low bone mass or osteoporosis, you should have your blood pressure checked while seated and again while standing to determine whether or not you have orthostatic hypotension. A drop in systolic blood pressure greater than or equal to twenty points, and a ten-point drop in diastolic pressure means that you have orthostatic hypotension. Otherwise, low blood pressure is generally not a problem.

If You Have Orthostatic Hypotension

- Get up slowly after sitting or lying down to reduce dizziness and the risk of falling. Ideally, you should rise slowly from a lying to a sitting position and wait a few minutes before standing. You should stand *only* when there is support available to prevent you from falling.
- Don't stay in bed because you feel dizzy; this will only perpetuate the problem. Rather, try the following prestanding exercises before getting out of bed in the morning.

  1. Sit up in bed, letting your feet hang over the side of the bed. Flex your feet up toward you five or six times. This exercise prevents blood from pooling in your feet by stimulating the veins in your calves to pump blood back up toward your heart.
  2. Tense and relax your abdominal muscles several times. This exercise also helps encourage blood flow from the lower extremities back toward the upper body.
  3. Tense the muscles in your hands and arms several times by making a fist. Or squeeze tennis balls with your hands. These isometric exercises are some of the most potent stimulators of blood pressure.

- Wear elasticized support hose to help keep blood from pooling to the legs and to help circulate blood back up toward the brain when you stand.
- Avoid alcohol, which can aggravate orthostatic hypotension.

- If hot baths, steam baths, saunas, and whirlpools make you feel dizzy, avoid them. Heat dilates the blood vessels in the skin and lowers your blood pressure.
- Drink plenty of fluids, particularly when flying on airlines, in hot weather, and when you have a diarrheal illness or the flu. These conditions can cause you to lose fluids and become dehydrated, which will make the problem worse.
- Try elevating the head of your bed by stacking books or two-inch-by-six-inch blocks under the legs of the bed.
- If you take one of the following medications associated with postural hypotension, ask your physician if you can switch to another medication that doesn't have this side effect.

If you take . . .	Ask about switching to . . .
Antihypertensive medications	
Diuretics; clonidine (Catapres); guanabenz (Wytensin); methyldopa (Aldomet); prazosin (Minipress); terazosin (Hytrin)	Calcium channel blockers; ACE inhibitors; beta-blockers; hydralazine (Apresazide, Apresoline, Hydra-Zide, Resorptine, Ser-Ap-Es)
Antidepressants	
Amitriptyline (Elavil, Endep, Etrafon, Limbitrol, Triavil); MAO inhibitors (Nardil,Parnate)	Desipramine Norpramin; Pertofrane nortriptyline (Pamelor, Ventyl)
Sedatives	
Chlorpromazine (Thorazine); thioridazine (Mellaril); trifluoperazine (Stelazine)	Haloperidol (Haldol); fluphenazine (Prolixin); beta-blockers

Your physician may also recommend that you use salt tablets (take these only under the supervision of your doctor, since excessive sodium can *increase* blood pressure in some susceptible people) or other medications that may help improve orthostatic hypotension.

In the future, as researchers learn more about the causes of hypertension, it may be possible to tailor treatment to the individual, allowing your doctor to prescribe just the right lifestyle modifications and medications to suit your needs. In the meantime, hypertension remains one of the most easily treatable of the major risk factors for heart disease and stroke. Keeping your blood pressure in check has been proven to reduce significantly your risk of having a heart attack or stroke. So if you have high blood pressure, don't ignore it or wait for it to go away. Get the treatment you need now, and if you need medication, use it every day.

CHAPTER 14

Stroke

STROKE IS A MAJOR CAUSE of disability and death among women in their middle and later years. But it doesn't have to be that way. Strokes *can* be prevented. In fact, the number of people who suffer a stroke has been declining for more than twenty years. The primary reason for this decline is a better understanding and management of the many risk factors for stroke by physicians and especially by people like you.

In addition, more and more people are surviving stroke today, and many are living productive lives, thanks to new and aggressive treatments for stroke and better programs for rehabilitation after stroke.

As with so many other preventable forms of cardiovascular disease, education is your first line of protection against stroke. Here is what you need to know to prevent a stroke, how to recognize the warning signs of stroke, and what to do if you or a loved one should have a stroke.

What Is a Stroke?

Generally speaking, a stroke occurs when the blood supply to the brain is disrupted. There are four main types of stroke (see Figure 13 on page 228):

Cerebral thrombosis. This is the most common type of stroke. It occurs when a blood clot (thrombus) forms and blocks blood flow in an artery supplying blood to part of the brain.

Cerebral embolism. This type of stroke occurs when a wandering clot (embolus) or some other particle forms in a blood vessel away from the brain (usually in the heart). The clot is carried by the bloodstream until it lodges in an artery leading to or in the brain.

Cerebral hemorrhage. This type of stroke occurs when an artery in the brain bursts, flooding the surrounding tissue with blood.

Subarachnoid hemorrhage. This type of stroke occurs when a blood vessel on the surface of the brain ruptures and bleeds into the space between the brain and the skull, but not into the brain itself.

The danger with any type of stroke is that whenever the blood supply to the brain is disrupted, brain tissue is deprived of oxygen and nutrients. If the disruption of blood flow lasts for too long, the brain tissue begins to die.

The damage and disability caused by stroke depend on which portion of the brain is affected. The right hemisphere of the brain controls the left side of the body, along with visual and spatial awareness. A stroke that occurs in this hemisphere of the brain can affect the ability to recognize shapes, angles, and proportions, as well as friends, family, or even parts of a stroke victim's own body. Musical ability may also be affected, since it, too, is governed by the right hemisphere.

The left hemisphere of the brain controls the right side of the body. It also controls analytical thought and problem-solving abilities. This hemisphere is usually thought of as the "logical" side of the brain. Damage to this portion of the brain can result in problems with language and mathematical abilities. The good news is that because the left and right hemispheres of the brain interact constantly, one side of the brain can sometimes learn to take on the tasks of another part of the brain that has been damaged by stroke.

Who Is at Risk?

Some people are at a greater risk of developing a stroke than others. How many of the following risk factors do you have?

Your Age

Everyone's risk of stroke increases with age. In fact, the incidence of stroke more than doubles in each successive decade after age sixty-five. The aging process itself, including "hardening of the arteries," makes the blood

FIGURE 13 — Four Types of Stroke

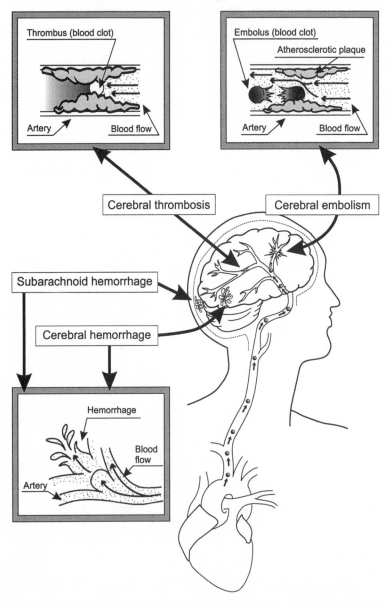

vessels more fragile and vulnerable to the development of blood clots or breakage.

In addition, some medical conditions tend to worsen with age, such as high blood pressure and diabetes, two major risk factors for stroke. So if you are over age sixty-five, you should consider yourself at an increased risk of having a stroke.

Your Gender
Women are 30 percent less likely to have a stroke than men. In spite of the lower incidence of stroke in women, however, more women than men die of stroke, accounting for more than 60 percent of deaths caused by stroke. It may be simply that women tend to live longer than men, and their older age increases the risk of dying from a stroke. Older women also have more risk factors for stroke.

Your Ethnic Background
For reasons that aren't clear, stroke is more prevalent among African-Americans than Caucasians. In fact, blacks are 60 percent more likely to have a stroke than whites. Black women are especially vulnerable. In 1990, for example, black women were 80 percent more likely to die from a stroke than white women.

African-Americans may be particularly at risk because they are also more likely to have many of the risk factors for stroke, including obesity, high blood pressure, diabetes, drinking problems, heart disease, cigarette smoking, and sickle-cell disease. In addition, genetic differences may account for some of the variability in the incidence of stroke among various ethnic groups.

A Family History of Stroke
If someone in your immediate family (a grandparent, parent, or sibling) has suffered a stroke, you should consider yourself at risk as well. A 1992 study of 9,475 male twins suggests that genes may strongly influence a person's risk of suffering a stroke. In that study, men with an identical twin who had a stroke were five times more likely to have a stroke themselves than men with a fraternal twin who had had a stroke. (Identical twins develop from the same fertilized egg and share the same genes, allowing scientists to distinguish genetic from environmental influences.)

Carotid Bruit
If you have an *asymptomatic carotid bruit* (an abnormal sound when a stethoscope is placed over the carotid artery in the neck), you are also at an increased risk of stroke. Make sure your physician listens to the carotid

artery in your neck; this vital part of your annual physical examination takes just a minute or two.

Diabetes
Diabetes makes you more susceptible to having a stroke, particularly if you are a woman. However, the more carefully the diabetes is controlled, the lower is the probability of stroke.

Hypertension
The risk of stroke rises as blood pressure rises. On the other hand, studies now show that reducing blood pressure *definitely* reduces the risk of stroke, making high blood pressure one of the most important modifiable risk factors for stroke.

Heart Disease
Various forms of heart disease—a previous heart attack, atherosclerosis, having an artificial heart value, congestive heart failure, rheumatic heart disease, congenital heart defects, and certain kinds of cardiac arrhythmias—are associated with an increased risk of stroke. People with these forms of heart disease are twice as likely to have a stroke as those with normally functioning hearts.

High Red Blood Cell Count
A marked or even moderate increase in the red blood cell count is a risk factor for stroke. No one knows exactly why this is so. One theory holds that the sheer number of red blood cells may cause blood flow to become more sluggish, particularly in the smaller capillaries, which may increase the likelihood of developing clots.

Transient Ischemic Attacks (TIAs)
About 10 percent of strokes are preceded by "little strokes," or transient ischemic attacks. TIAs occur when a blood clot temporarily clogs an artery and part of the brain doesn't get the blood it needs. Symptoms include temporary weakness, clumsiness, or loss of feeling in an arm, leg, or the side of the face, temporary loss of vision in one eye, temporary loss of speech or difficulty speaking, and sometimes dizziness, double vision, and staggering.

Symptoms generally don't last long. More than 75 percent of TIAs last less than five minutes. However, TIAs can last up to twenty-four hours (although this is very unusual). Unlike stroke, when a TIA is over, people return to normal.

Cigarette Smoking

Cigarette smoking makes women especially vulnerable to stroke: Women who smoke have a 60 percent greater chance of having a debilitating stroke than those who don't. (Among men who smoke, the risk is 40 percent greater than among men who don't.) Women who smoke and also take oral contraceptives are at greatest risk. These women are twenty-two times more likely to have a stroke than women who don't smoke and who use other forms of contraception.

Heavy Alcohol Consumption

Heavy drinking and binge drinking appear to be strongly related to an increased risk of stroke. One reason may be that having more than two alcoholic beverages a day raises blood pressure, and high blood pressure is a significant risk factor for stroke.

Obesity

Being more than 30 percent overweight—the medical definition of obesity—can indirectly raise your risk of having a stroke by increasing your chances of developing hypertension, diabetes, and heart disease, three major risk factors for stroke.

Women are especially susceptible to developing these conditions if they are overweight. The risk is even greater for black women who are obese.

Drug Abuse

Stroke is a common result of abusing drugs. Particularly dangerous are stimulants such as cocaine and amphetamines, which raise blood pressure and blood flow very suddenly, sometimes causing small arteries in the brain to rupture as a result. If an aneurysm (a weak spot in an artery) is present or if there is an abnormality in the arteries, the increase in stroke risk is significant.

Overuse of Aspirin

Aspirin is often prescribed to help prevent an embolic stroke (a stroke caused by a blood clot) in certain people who are at a high risk of having one, including those with a high red blood cell count, those with existing coronary artery disease, those with atrial fibrillation (a specific kind of abnormal heart rhythm), those who have had TIAs, and those with artificial heart valves. However, overuse of aspirin can actually trigger a hemorrhagic stroke. For this reason, you should *not* take aspirin every day for stroke prevention unless your doctor recommends it. (For more on aspirin's use in the prevention of stroke, see page 235.)

WHAT ABOUT ESTROGEN?

Many women worry about taking estrogen (either in the form of oral contraceptives or postmenopausal estrogen therapy) for fear the hormones cause blood clots that can trigger a stroke. Is it true that estrogen causes blood clots? Let's take a closer look at the evidence for both forms of estrogen.

ORAL CONTRACEPTIVES. Some early studies involving oral contraceptives containing large doses of the hormones estrogen and progestogen did find an increased risk of stroke among women who used them. But at least one of the major studies during the 1970s was flawed because it failed to take into account women who smoked cigarettes. When these women were excluded from the study, researchers found that oral contraceptives were associated with only a slight increase in stroke risk, mainly among women over age forty.

Today's oral contraceptives contain much lower doses of estrogen and progestogen, and more recent studies (including our own) have found that the new low-dose oral contraceptives appear to have a minimal effect on the development of venous thrombosis (blood clots in the veins). Occasionally, however, women taking oral contraceptives will develop a more dangerous arterial blood clot. No one fully understands why this is so. We recommend that older women (over age thirty-five) who take birth control pills also take a junior aspirin (60 milligrams) once every three days to help reduce the risk of a blood clot forming.

As for hypertension, only a very small percentage of women (5 percent) will develop high blood pressure while taking oral contraceptives. Usually, blood pressure returns to normal again after you stop taking birth control pills.

One thing is clear: If you smoke cigarettes and take oral

contraceptives, your risk of having a stroke skyrockets. If you can't seem to quit smoking, you should use another form of contraception. (For more on oral contraceptives and cardiovascular risk, see Chapter 9.)

POSTMENOPAUSAL ESTROGENS. Postmenopausal hormones developed a bad reputation mostly by association with the early studies on oral contraceptives, which found an increased risk of blood clots, heart attacks, and strokes among users. More recent studies have found that postmenopausal hormone therapy is not associated with an increased risk of having a stroke, and may actually reduce the risk of embolic stroke.

In one study, postmenopausal estrogens were found to reduce the "stickiness" of platelets. In another, women who took postmenopausal estrogens had lower levels of a blood coagulant known as Factor VII, compared with women who didn't take estrogen. Moreover, natural estrogens *don't* reduce blood levels of antithrombin III, a potent anticoagulant that is a good marker for predicting whether or not a blood clot will develop. And in the PEPI Trial (see page 157) women who took both estrogen and progestogen had lower levels of the blood coagulant fibrinogen than women who took estrogen alone or no hormones at all.

And while oral estrogens are known to raise the levels of several blood proteins involved in coagulation, these are not biologically active until they're exposed to an injured blood vessel. Plus, "normal" levels of these proteins vary widely, and are not useful markers for predicting your risk of developing a blood clot.

The bottom line is that no study shows a cause-and-effect relationship between taking postmenopausal estrogens and the development of blood clots.

How to Prevent a Stroke

The best way to prevent a stroke (as well as a host of other health problems) is to reduce or eliminate all of the risk factors for stroke that you can. Of course, some risk factors, such as your age and gender, cannot be changed.

But many of the most important risk factors for stroke can be influenced. Here are some of the more important ways you can reduce your risk of having a stroke.

If You Smoke, Quit

There isn't much good that can be said about cigarette smoking, except that if you quit, your risk of stroke (along with other health hazards associated with smoking) begins to decline. The Nurses' Health Study, begun in 1976, following 117,006 female registered nurses for twelve years, found that women who quit smoking for less than two years reduced their risk of stroke by 22 percent. Two to four years after quitting, their risk returned to that of women who had never smoked. (For tips on quitting, see Chapter 8.)

Control High Blood Pressure

Have your blood pressure checked regularly. If it is high, be sure to follow your doctor's advice carefully for keeping high blood pressure under control: follow a low-salt diet, exercise regularly, drink alcohol in moderation, and maintain a healthy weight. If you take antihypertensive medication, be sure to take it every day. (For more on preventing and treating high blood pressure, see Chapter 13.)

Keep Diabetes in Check

This usually means working closely with your doctor and a registered dietitian to keep your blood sugar levels normal. Most people have Type II, or non-insulin-dependent, diabetes, a form of diabetes that can often be controlled with a healthy low-fat diet, regular moderate exercise, and (most important of all) weight loss.

Lower Your Blood Cholesterol Levels

Coronary artery disease, a significant risk factor for stroke, can be prevented, in part by keeping a close watch on your blood cholesterol levels. Have your doctor periodically check your blood cholesterol levels (see page 67). If they are high, follow the guidelines for lowering them and for reducing your risk of coronary artery disease in Part II of this book.

Drink Alcohol in Moderation

Having as little as three drinks per day can raise your blood pressure, and can thwart any efforts at lowering your blood pressure if you already have hypertension. Since hypertension is a major risk factor for stroke, you should limit the amount of alcohol you consume to no more than two drinks per day. (One drink contains the equivalent of 1 ounce of 100-proof spirits, 1.5 ounces of 80-proof spirits, 4 ounces of wine, or 12 ounces of beer.)

Exercise Regularly

A program of regular moderate physical activity helps lower blood pressure, increases levels of protective HDL cholesterol, helps control weight problems, and reduces your risk of having a heart attack or stroke. (For more on beginning an exercise program, see Chapter 7. If you already have heart disease, use the exercise guidelines on page 127.)

Maintain a Healthy Weight

Keeping your weight in check will reduce your risk of developing hypertension, atherosclerosis, and diabetes, all major risk factors for stroke. A low-fat diet combined with a regular exercise program is the best way to lose weight and keep the weight off. You may be more likely to succeed if you work closely with your physician and a registered dietition. (For more on weight loss, see page 139.)

Use Aspirin Judiciously

Use aspirin only on the advice and guidance of your physician. If you have a high red blood cell count, have had TIAs, or have coronary artery disease, your physician may recommend that you take aspirin to help prevent the formation of a clot. But because overuse of aspirin has been associated with an increased risk of hemorrhagic stroke, be sure to take aspirin only with your physician's knowledge and on his or her recommendation.

Seek Medical Help for TIAS

Promptly see your doctor if you develop symptoms of TIAs. These include temporary weakness; clumsiness or loss of feeling in an arm, leg, or the side of the face; temporary loss of vision in one eye; temporary loss of speech or difficulty speaking; and sometimes dizziness, double vision, and staggering. Your doctor can help determine whether or not you've had a TIA or whether the symptoms arose from another condition.

If You or a Loved One Has a Stroke

Until recently, if you or a loved one developed the symptoms of a stroke, you might not have been treated by a doctor until the next day. Many doctors thought that early intervention would do nothing to halt a stroke or change its outcome. Doctors now believe that the sooner a stroke is treated and blood flow restored, the better the prognosis.

The National Stroke Association has issued universal guidelines that support a "six-hour window," a critical time during which a stroke should be evaluated and treated. This change in recommendations is evidenced by the phrase "brain attack." If someone has a heart attack, doctors perform all manner of life-saving techniques to reduce or even reverse the damage. By calling strokes "brain attacks" the National Stroke Association hopes people will recognize that stroke needs immediate medical attention.

Warning Signs of a Stroke

Unfortunately, studies have found that fewer than 30 percent of patients know the warning signs of stroke or realize that the symptoms they have are caused by a stroke. Do you?

- Sudden weakness or numbness of the face, arm, or leg on one side of the body
- Sudden dimness or loss of vision, particularly in one eye
- Loss of speech, or trouble talking or understanding speech
- Sudden severe headaches with no apparent cause
- Unexplained dizziness, unsteadiness, or sudden falls, especially along with any of the previous symptoms

Making a Diagnosis

If you develop any of the symptoms of stroke, you should seek medical attention within six hours of their onset. The sooner you get medical attention, the more likely you will be to survive a stroke and to minimize damage to brain tissue.

If you go to a hospital emergency room, you will likely be evaluated and treated by an emergency brain resuscitation (EBR) team. These are medical personnel who have been specially trained in rapid diagnosis and treatment of stroke patients.

The EBR team will first check your breathing to ensure that airways are clear. The team will also check your temperature, blood pressure, and other vital signs. Urine and blood tests will be administered to determine if any chemical abnormalities or imbalances may have contributed to the stroke. (High cholesterol levels, for example, may indicate the presence of significant atherosclerosis. Blood in the urine may indicate the stroke has been caused by an embolus.)

If your blood pressure is high, your physician will try to bring it down slowly in order to prevent further damage to oxygen-starved brain tissue.

Your physician will want to know your personal and family medical history, as well as any medications you may be taking. (A family member or close friend may have to assist you if your speech has been impaired by the stroke.) You may also have to have an electrocardiogram (ECG) to determine whether or not you also have heart disease, which is often a cause of stroke.

The medical team will take your pulse at various places around the body, particularly the carotid artery in the neck. Comparing the different pulses helps identify the location of the stroke-affected area.

A neurological examination will be performed to assist in locating the area of stroke, as well as to determine the extent of damage that may have already occurred. The evaluation may include a number of "spot tests," such as asking you where you are to determine your sense of orientation. You may be asked to walk a few steps, or to move your arms and legs. Eye movement and vision will be checked as well.

You may also undergo a computed tomography (CT) scan of the brain. This is a fast and painless X-ray examination that creates a three-dimensional image of the brain. It is one of the best ways to determine if the stroke was due to bleeding (hemorrhage) or blockage (ischemia).

Many hospitals now also offer magnetic resonance imaging (MRI), the use of a strong magnetic field and radio waves to generate a three-dimensional image of the brain without radiation exposure. Both bleeding and blockage are easily identified through the use of MRIs. A related test, known as magnetic resonance angiography (MRA), can be used to create three-dimensional images of veins and arteries in both the neck and the brain.

Ultrasound testing may be used to determine the extent and location of damage in an artery, as well as to collect information on blood flow, which can be critical to deciding what kind of treatment you need.

Sometimes more invasive procedures are required. The two most commonly used are lumbar puncture (also known as a spinal tap) and angiography. A lumbar puncture gives the physician access to the cerebrospinal fluid, the liquid that cushions the brain. This procedure can determine if the stroke was hemorrhagic or caused by a blood clot.

Angiography is used to evaluate the size and location of blockages in the neck and intracranial blood vessels. The procedure involves inserting a catheter into an artery and injecting dyes into the blood vessels. These dyes illuminate the vessels and make any blockages visible on X rays.

How Strokes Are Treated

Once the medical team has determined the specific area of the brain in which the stroke occurred and the severity of the damage, proper treatment and rehabilitation can begin.

Treatment in the hospital after a stroke varies, depending on the cause of the stroke, the overall condition of the patient, and the degree of damage the stroke has caused.

If the cause of the stroke is atherosclerosis damage to the carotid arteries, which run up along the front of the neck, a surgical procedure known as *carotid endarterectomy* may be required to remove plaques that have formed along an artery's inner lining (see Figure 14). A less invasive procedure, known as *angioplasty*, involves the use of a small device, typically a balloon, that is inserted into the blocked blood vessel through a catheter. The device is then inflated or expanded to pry open the passage and restore blood flow. (See 193 and pages following for a complete discussion of angioplasty.)

Treatment of the blood with a variety of drugs can sometimes improve blood flow to the brain. Three main types of drugs are used to prevent the formation of blood clots and/or dissolve existing clots in the blood vessels: *antiplatelet* drugs, *anticoagulant* drugs, and *thrombolytic* drugs. Each type of drug interferes with a different step in the blood-clotting process.

Antiplatelet drugs include *aspirin, dipyridamole* (brand name Persantine), *sulfinpyrazone* (brand name Anturane), and *ticlopidine* (brand name Ticlid). These drugs help keep platelets from sticking together—the first step in the formation of a blood clot. They are often prescribed to prevent blood clots from forming in people with existing coronary artery disease, those with artificial heart valves or atrial fibrillation, and those who have previously had TIAs or strokes.

Anticoagulant drugs, including *heparin* and *warfarin*, help maintain blood flow, prevent an existing clot from getting bigger, and can prevent clots from forming inside the arteries and veins. Heparin, given by injection, works by preventing the formation of a clot-forming substance known as *thrombin* in the blood. Heparin takes effect immediately. Warfarin, given in the form of a pill, interferes with the formation of certain blood-clotting factors manufactured by the liver. It also blocks the action of vitamin K, which plays a role in the formation of blood clots. Warfarin must be taken for several days to become effective.

Antithrombotic drugs, including *streptokinase, tissue-plasminogen activator, urokinase,* and *anistreplase,* are used to dissolve existing clots. The drugs are usually given intravenously or directly into an obstructed artery

FIGURE 14 — Carotid Endarterectomy

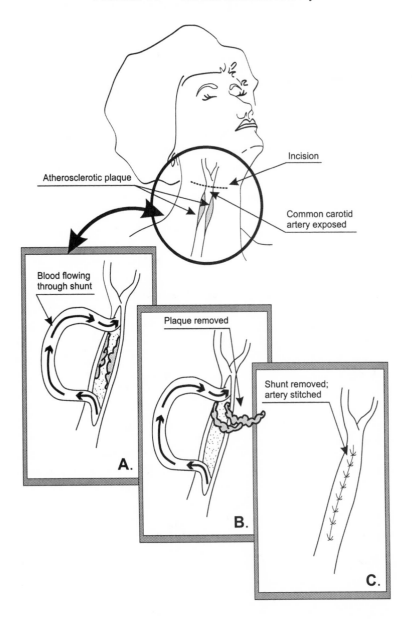

Incision

Atherosclerotic plaque

Common carotid artery exposed

Blood flowing through shunt

Plaque removed

Shunt removed; artery stitched

A.

B.

C.

or vein. They work by increasing blood levels of plasmin, an enzyme that breaks up the tough fibrin strands that hold a clot together.

In some cases of stroke, hematomas or pools of blood may form in the brain due to bleeding. Hematomas can create pressure on the brain that causes brain tissue to die. It may be necessary in these cases to drain the fluid from the brain surgically.

Recovery and Rehabilitation

Rehabilitation is a key part of recovering from a stroke. Typically, a rehabilitation team for a stroke survivor includes a variety of professionals, as well as the family. Some of the professionals who may be involved include the primary physician, medical specialists (neurologists, cardiologists, etc.), a dietitian/nutritionist, a rehabilitation nurse, a physical therapist, an occupational therapist, a vocational therapist, a speech therapist, a recreational therapist, a social worker, and a psychologist. Not every patient will need all of these, and most will need only a few of the specialty therapists. All patients, however, will require the attention and care of the family.

In the first few days or weeks after a stroke, the primary goal of rehabilitation is to prevent joints and muscles in any paralyzed limbs from contracting. In the weeks following the stroke, recovery varies widely, with some patients showing marked improvement in movement, speech, vision, and sensory perception and others making slower progress.

Patients are encouraged, if possible, to get out of bed a day or two after suffering a stroke. Those with complicating medical conditions, such as diabetes or heart disease, may have to remain in bed for up to five days.

Physical therapy evaluates the level of physical disability and the degree of recovery that can be expected. Physical therapists start patients on "range-of-motion" exercises designed to prevent pain and stiffness from developing in joints. Later more demanding physical therapies are introduced to assist the patient in regaining mobility and use of paralyzed limbs, although this may be limited in some patients.

Occupational therapy is primarily concerned with the upper body of the stroke patient. The occupational therapist will concentrate on helping the stroke survivor rehabilitate practical skills that are needed at home or on the job.

Speech therapy is commonly required in stroke rehabilitation. Difficulties with speech and language appear in stroke survivors with right arm and leg weakness. Occasionally stroke in the brain stem affects speech. After three months, most stroke survivors' speech recovery stabilizes. At this point the goal becomes to maximize the patient's remaining language function. Strategies for this will vary depending on the patient's condition and personality. Some patients with left brain damage can learn to "sing" the words they need due to the musical ability of the right brain. Others may require word boards or boards that contain short phrases to which the patient can point. There are also electronic word boards, which may be easier for some stroke survivors to use.

Returning Home After a Stroke

The majority of stroke patients are able to return to their homes and resume many of their former activities. Others must change their living arrangements.

A nursing facility may be an essential transitional step for a bedridden stroke survivor. Skilled nursing facilities provide twenty-four-hour care, as well as frequent monitoring by a physician. Nursing facilities also allow a greater opportunity for therapy, and allow the family time to ready the home for the return of a person with special needs.

Intermediate-care facilities are the preferred choice for patients who are more independent and have no serious medical problems. These facilities generally provide nursing care during the day, twenty-four-hour supervision, and social activities.

Stroke survivors who are able to return to their homes, but who live alone, should follow a few simple rules to ensure greater safety in the event of a recurrent stroke incident. These are:

- Arrange for someone to call the home at least once a day.
- Develop a signal system with neighbors that will alert them to potential problems, particularly if you are not able to speak.
- Let the local fire department know of your condition. Give your name, address, and phone number and other information so that they may be better able to assist in an emergency.
- Talk to the postmaster or the mail carrier about enrolling in the U.S. Postal Alert program. This program has an identifying sticker that is placed on the mailbox. If mail accumulates, the carrier can notify an appropriate agency or service.

Family members should assess the home for any changes required in order to make it accessible to the patient. Items to keep in mind are steps, slope to driveways and yards, the proximity of parking to the house, lighting, and handrails. Inside the house leave plenty of room for the patient to maneuver around furniture, check to see that doorways are wide enough for wheelchairs, make sure the flooring, tubs, and showers have nonskid surfaces, and that the home is equipped with safety equipment (telephones, fire extinguishers, smoke detectors).

Much has been learned about stroke in the last twenty years. The death rate from stroke has fallen to 50 percent of what it was twenty-two years ago. With three million stroke survivors in this country, there is obvious reason for optimism regarding treatment and rehabilitation after stroke.

Most important is the knowledge that stroke can be prevented, or the risks at least lessened, by making healthy lifestyle choices.

THE STROKE CONNECTION NETWORK

Stroke survivors and their families face a major challenge in coping with the sudden and abrupt changes caused by stroke. Living arrangements, careers, and relationships are often altered by the damage resulting from stroke.

The American Heart Association has a program called the "Stroke Connection Network." The network provides services to stroke survivors and their families, and gives them the opportunity to relate to other people with similar problems. These "stroke clubs" reduce the loneliness, increase the coping skills, and provide assistance for dealing with stroke.

The services provided by the Stroke Connection Network include:

- *Stroke Connection*, a newsletter that provides information on stroke, coping, and real-life experiences from members
- *Stroke of Luck*, an informal newsletter for people with aphasia, a communication disorder commonly caused by stroke
- Educational materials for stroke patients and their families
- A toll-free, long-distance number to answer stroke questions. The number is 1-800-553-6321.

CHAPTER 15

Other Cardiovascular Conditions

ALTHOUGH CORONARY ARTERY DISEASE is one of the most common causes of heart trouble in women, it is by no means the only one. Here's what you need to know about a few other heart conditions that commonly affect women.

Arrhythmias

You've undoubtedly experienced it at some point in your life: a pounding sensation in your chest or a feeling that your heart is racing. Or perhaps you've felt occasionally that your heart skipped a beat. These are known as *arrhythmias*, irregularities in the heart's rate or rhythm. Generally speaking, arrhythmias occur when the heart's natural pacemaker, the sinoatrial node, develops an abnormal rate or rhythm, when the normal pathway of electrical current is interrupted, or when another part of the heart takes over as pacemaker. (For more on the SA node and the electrical system of the heart, see "How Your Heart Beats," on page 244).

If you do not already have heart disease, the occasional "skipped beat" or racing heart, particularly just before or after an anxiety-producing situation or after one-too-many cups of coffee, are usually harmless and nothing to worry about. If you suffer from menopausal hot flashes, you may experience a pounding or racing heart with every hot flash. Again, while the feeling can be uncomfortable, it is rarely life threatening.

That's not to say that *all* heartbeat irregularities are to be tossed off as

HOW YOUR HEART BEATS

Your heart pumps blood to the lungs and all of your body's tissues through a sequence of highly organized contractions of its four chambers and four valves. Heartbeats are governed by an electrical impulse that originates in a pea-sized bundle of highly specialized cells known as the *sinoatrial node* (SA node), the heart's natural pacemaker. The sinoatrial node is located in the upper-right chamber (atrium) of the heart (see Figure 15.)

The SA node fires off electrical impulses about once every second when the heart is at rest. From the SA node, the electrical impulses travel through three bundles of specialized tissues down to the atrioventricular (AV) node. As the electrical impulses travel to the AV node, some of them fan out through the left and right atria, causing the two upper chambers to contract while the lower chambers fill with blood.

The AV node acts as a relay station, carrying the electrical impulses to the lower (ventricular) heart chambers. The impulses travel rapidly through the lower chambers in what are known as the left and right bundle branches, causing the lower chambers to contract simultaneously.

Two major types of nerves also travel to the heart and can influence the sinus node: the sympathetic nervous system and the parasympathetic nervous system (also known as the vagal nervous system). The sympathetic nervous system can speed up the heart rate and the parasympathetic nervous system can slow it down. Hormones, such as epinephrine, can also influence your heart rate. This is why your heart often starts to pound when you are startled.

harmless. Some, in fact, can be life threatening and require immediate medical attention, especially if you have existing heart problems.

How can you tell harmless arrhythmias from life-threatening ones? *Any recurring or persistent heartbeat irregularities or abnormal heart rhythms, especially those accompanied by chest discomfort, dizziness, or fainting, should promptly be brought to the attention of your doctor, even if you think they're harmless.* Your physician can properly evaluate your condition, first by listening to your heart with a stethoscope. If necessary, you may have to have an electrocardiogram (ECG) (see page 72). If the

FIGURE 15 — The Sinoatrial Node and the Heart's Conduction System

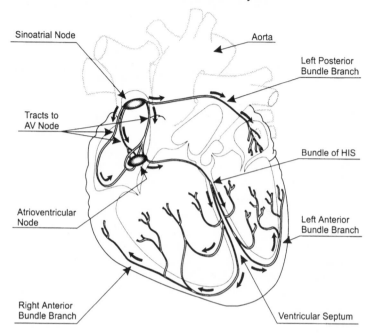

abnormal rhythm occurs intermittently, you may have to wear a Holter monitor for twenty-four hours (see page 77) as you go about your normal activities. An echocardiogram may also be required to determine whether the heart itself is damaged or diseased.

There are several types of rhythm disturbances that you should be aware of. These include the following:

Tachycardia

Tachycardia is a rapid heartbeat above ninety to one hundred beats per minute. Tachycardia may last just a few seconds or up to several hours. The rapid heartbeat may stop as suddenly as it began or it may gradually slow to a level below ninety beats per minute. You may experience such symptoms as a rapid pulse, heart palpitations, or a pounding sensation in the chest. Sometimes, the pounding sensation may extend into the throat or head.

There are actually two types of rapid heartbeat. *Sinus tachycardia* occurs when the upper chambers of the heart beat too fast; it is characterized by a gradual rise in your heart rate to over one hundred beats per minute. Typically, sinus tachycardia occurs when excitement, stress, or physical activity causes the adrenal glands to release the "stress" hormone epinephrine, stimulating the sinus node and speeding up the heart rate. Thyroid problems and menopausal hot flashes may also trigger bouts of sinus tachycardia.

Another type of tachycardia, known as *paroxysmal atrial tachycardia* (PAT) is characterized by a sudden jump in the heart rate to between 150 and 170 beats per minute.

Both types of tachycardia are bothersome but are generally harmless unless you have existing coronary artery disease, congestive heart failure, or other serious forms of heart disease. If you have coronary artery disease, rapid heartbeats can trigger painful bouts of angina.

Treatment of sinus tachycardia is fairly simple: Identifying and treating the underlying cause usually resolves the problem. Paroxysmal atrial tachycardia, on the other hand, often requires treatment with drugs. Your doctor may prescribe Digoxin, a beta-blocker, or a combination of these drugs. Often, after about two or three months of treatment, the episodes occur less frequently or stop altogether, and you may be able to stop drug therapy altogether or use your prescribed medication only when needed.

Atrial Fibrillation

This condition (also known as flutter) occurs when the heart's upper chambers begin to beat rapidly and irregularly, causing the lower chambers to beat irregularly, too. Symptoms include heart palpitations and a pounding sensation in the chest. Atrial fibrillation may sometimes cause you to feel lightheaded or pass out.

You may develop atrial fibrillation if you have coronary artery disease, severe, longstanding hypertension, mitral valve prolapse, or an overactive thyroid gland (hyperthyroidism). But even people with a normal, healthy heart sometimes develop atrial fibrillation.

If the condition is diagnosed within a few days or a week after you develop it, it can often be effectively treated with drugs—usually digitalis (Digoxin). If Digoxin doesn't help, other drugs may be used, including calcium channel blockers, beta-blockers, procainamide, disopyramide, or quinidine.

If you have had the problem for several weeks or months, your doctor may first prescribe anticoagulants, such as warfarin, for several weeks before treating the arrhythmia. This is because there is a slight chance that a blood clot will form in the left atrium or the mitral valve, and that can break free when the heart converts back to a normal rhythm. Anticoagulants help break up any blood clots that may have already formed, and prevent new blood clots from forming.

If the arrhythmia doesn't respond to drug therapy, it may be necessary for you to be treated in the hospital with electric cardioversion. During the procedure, you will be given an intravenous anesthetic that puts you to sleep for just a few moments. While you are asleep, your doctor will apply an electric shock to the chest. This usually converts the heart to a normal rhythm.

Premature Beats, Ventricular Arrhythmia, and Ventricular Fibrillation

These types of arrhythmia don't originate in the sinus node, but arise from elsewhere in the heart. When they occur in the upper chambers of the heart, these abnormal heart rhythms are known as *premature atrial contractions* (PACs); when they originate in the lower chambers, they are known as *premature ventricular contractions* (PVCs).

Although PACs can be irritating, they are usually harmless and don't require any treatment. Unfortunately, the same cannot be said about all premature ventricular contractions. PVCs come in two forms: benign and malignant. Many perfectly healthy people have occasional benign PVCs and feel as though their hearts skipped a beat. These are usually harmless and can be triggered by fatigue, cigarette smoking, caffeine-containing beverages or other stimulants, or excessive amounts of alcohol. Viral infections that inflame the heart (slightly) can also cause these premature beats, as can elevated levels of thyroid hormone and certain medications, such as the asthma medication theophylline.

Malignant PVCs, on the other hand, can be life threatening. These premature beats usually occur in people with existing heart disease, including coronary artery disease, valve disease, or *cardiomyopathy* (a thickening of the heart muscle that causes it to pump blood less efficiently). Malignant PVCs can also be triggered by a heart attack.

If the heartbeats are very rapid, PVCs can cause you to faint and regain consciousness after several seconds or minutes, once the heart returns to a normal rhythm. Occasionally, however, a series of PVCs can develop into ventricular fibrillation, in which the lower chambers of the heart quiver uncontrollably. *This is a life-threatening medical emergency because the heart can no longer beat or pump blood effectively.* Ventricular fibrillation must be promptly treated with cardiopulmonary resuscitation (CPR) or cardioversion (electroshock treatments to the heart).

Fortunately, most people have benign premature beats. If your heart is otherwise healthy and you are diagnosed with premature beats, you and your doctor should work together to pinpoint and treat the underlying cause of the premature beats, which usually resolves the problem.

What about malignant PVCs? If you have mild coronary artery disease and occasional bouts of ventricular arrhythmias, all that may be needed is to treat the underlying heart disease (with diet, exercise, drugs, or possibly balloon angioplasty). For the most part, however, malignant PVCs require aggressive treatment, especially if you have previously developed ventricular arrhythmias or ventricular fibrillation.

Your doctor may first recommend that you eliminate any stimulants that may aggravate your condition, such as caffeine or nicotine. He or she will also review the medications you take to determine whether any of them may be contributing to the problem. You will also likely be prescribed one or more antiarrhythmic medications, including beta-blockers, calcium channel blockers, and other antiarrhythmic drugs, such as procainamide, lidocaine, quinidine, mexiletine, and disopyramide.

If you have serious rhythm disturbances that don't respond to lifestyle changes and medication, there are two fairly new treatment options that may be available to you. One involves implantation of a special pacemaker called an *internal defibrillator*. The only time the defibrillator is activated is when you have an episode of ventricular tachycardia or ventricular fibrillation. The defibrillator administers an electric shock to the heart, which returns the heart to a normal rhythm.

The other is a highly specialized type of surgery that involves removing the portion of the heart tissue that is triggering the episodes. During the operation, the surgeon uses a specialized computer to determine which part of the heart is causing the problem. The heart tissue in that area is then removed.

Heart Block

This term refers to a slowdown in the passage of electrical currents through the heart. Some forms of heart block are not serious. They may sometimes cause a slight slowdown of heartbeats (known as *bradycardia*), but often don't cause any symptoms at all. The most serious is third-degree heart block, also known as complete heart block. This type of heart block occurs when the electrical impulses generated in the upper chambers are completely blocked from traveling the lower chambers, causing a serious slowing of heartbeats in the ventricular chambers (less than 40 beats per minute).

The main symptom of complete heart block is fainting or near-fainting spells. The condition must usually be treated with an artificial pacemaker.

Mitral Valve Prolapse and Other Problems with the Heart Valves

The heart has four valves: the *aortic valve*, the *pulmonary valve*, the *tricuspid valve*, and the *mitral valve*. Their main purpose is to help control the flow of blood through the heart's four chambers, and to make sure it always flows in the right direction.

Unlike the heart, which is composed of muscle tissue, the valves are made of a tough fibrous tissue similar to the ligaments in your joints. They are covered with a thin layer of cells known as *endocardium*.

Diseases of the heart valves usually involve one or two basic problems: *valvular stenosis* occurs when a diseased valve thickens, becomes scarred, and develops calcium deposits. This thickening and scarring narrows the passage through which blood can flow, interfering with the normal flow of blood through the heart's chambers. *Valvular regurgitation* occurs when scarring and calcium deposits on a valve keep it from closing properly, allowing blood to flow back into the chamber from which it is being pumped. A woman with valvular heart disease can develop one or the other of these problems, or have both at the same time.

Valvular heart disease can have any of a number of causes. Some women are born with defective valves, which can, over time, become scarred and develop calcium deposits. In the past, rheumatic fever, which develops when a strep throat is not properly treated with antibiotics, was a common cause of valve problems, as was syphilis, a sexually transmitted disease. If you already have a diseased heart valve, you are more vulnerable to developing endocarditis, a bacterial infection of the thin layer of cells covering the heart valve. Endocarditis can cause more scarring and thickening of an already diseased valve.

Any of the heart's four valves can develop problems. But the most common valvular problem—especially for women—is mitral valve prolapse.

Mitral valve prolapse (MVP) occurs when one or both leaflets that make up the mitral valve billow up into the heart's atrial chamber, often resulting in a clicking sound, or heart murmur (see Figure 16). The condition sometimes causes blood to be spilled back into the atrium, a condition known as *regurgitation*.

For reasons unknown, MVP is more common in women than men, affecting about 5 to 6 percent of women, compared to 2 to 3 percent of men. There are two types: patients with Type I MVP have no other heart abnormalities, only slight thickening of the mitral valve, and mild regurgitation. Those with Type II MVP, the more serious form, often develop abnormalities of the valve itself, severe thickening, and increased regurgitation of blood.

Chest pain is the most frequent symptom, occurring in as many as 50 to 60 percent of women with MVP. Palpitations, chronic fatigue, and a feeling of anxiety are common too. Some women experience shortness of breath and/or dizzy spells. Only rarely, however, does MVP lead to more serious heart problems.

Your physician may be able to diagnose MVP simply by listening for the characteristic heart murmur that accompanies the condition. Your doctor can determine the severity of the condition with the help of an echocardiogram, in which sound waves are used to view the mitral valve in motion.

While symptoms may be bothersome, most women—particularly those with Type I MVP—won't require any treatment at all. If chest pain and palpitations are particularly bothersome to you, you should try to avoid nicotine, caffeine, and alcohol, all of which can aggravate these symptoms.

Some women with severe MVP may be advised to take a large dose of antibiotics an hour before having extensive dental work or surgery and again six hours later. This precaution is meant to help protect against *bacterial endocarditis*, an infection caused by bacteria circulating in the bloodstream that may become attached to the prolapsed mitral valve.

If mitral valve prolapse or other valve problems become severe, causing chronic chest pain, dizziness, or congestive heart failure, your doctor may recommend that you undergo further diagnostic tests, including an echocardiogram, a heart scan, and possibly cardiac catheterization, to see if you are a candidate for surgery. Some women with severe stenosis or obstruction of the mitral valve may benefit from a surgical procedure known as *valvuloplasty*, in which the surgeon's finger, a surgical instrument, or a catheter is used to widen the opening of the valve. Others, especially those with congestive heart failure, may require surgical replacement of the diseased valve with an artificial valve.

FIGURE 16 — Mitral Valve Prolapse

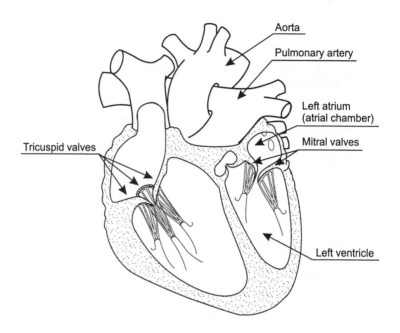

Aorta

Pulmonary artery

Left atrium
(atrial chamber)

Mitral valves

Tricuspid valves

Left ventricle

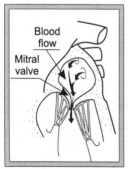

Blood
flow

Mitral
valve

Normal

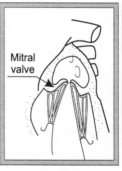

Mitral
valve

Mitral valve
prolapse

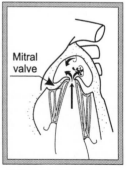

Mitral
valve

Mitral valve prolapse
with regurgitation

Congenital Heart Defects

Congenital heart defects are physical deformities of the heart that are present at birth. They occur in about five to ten of every one thousand live births. Without treatment, the majority of these people would die in infancy or childhood. But thanks to advances in the surgical repair of congenital heart defects, beginning as early as 1939 and continuing into the 1990s, most people born with these problems now can expect to survive into adolescence and adulthood. Indeed, in the U.S. alone, more than half a million men and women with serious congenital defects have reached adulthood over the past thirty years.

Although more patients are surviving, most defects are not totally corrected at birth. Many men and women must have repeat surgery as they grow older. Others, with mild heart defects that were well tolerated during childhood, may need their first operation as adults. So, in effect, if you have a congenital heart defect, you will require long-term surveillance and special care for as long as you live.

There are a number of different kinds of congenital defects, and a discussion of individual defects and their treatment is beyond the scope of this book. But here you will find some general guidelines for the medical care you can expect to receive, as well as some specific considerations for you as a woman.

Medical Complications

Some of the most common medical problems you may have to cope with if you have congenital heart disease include the following:

Arrhythmias. These are abnormal heart rhythms or disturbances in the electrical conduction system that governs heartbeats. Arrhythmias may develop for any of a number of reasons, including lack of sleep, too much caffeine, cigarette smoking, and excessive amounts of alcohol. The only difference is that rhythm disturbances that are usually harmless in people with a normal heart could be life threatening in people with congenital heart disease. For this reason, you should discuss with your doctor a plan for dealing with abnormal heart rhythms—*before* they develop. Your plan will undoubtedly involve such preventive measures as getting plenty of rest, and avoiding caffeine, cigarettes, and alcohol. If you do happen to develop arrhythmias, there are a number of highly effective medications that can be used to treat them. (For more on antiarrhythmic medications, see page 184.)

Infective endocarditis. Whether or not you have a defect that has been surgically repaired, you are at a greater risk for developing infective endocarditis, an infection of the membrane lining the inside of the heart and the heart valves. The condition is usually caused by a bacterial infection in another part of the body. Symptoms include fever, malaise, and possibly changes in heart rhythms. The danger is that the heart valves may become damaged.

To prevent infective endocarditis, you will be advised to take prophylactic antibiotics whenever you undergo an invasive medical procedure, including dental work, certain gynecological procedures, cardiac catheterization, transesophageal echocardiography (in which a miniature ultrasound probe is inserted through your esophagus) and any time you have surgery. Even having your ears (or other body parts) pierced, or getting a tattoo puts you at risk and requires prophylactic antibiotics. In addition, you should always carry a medical ID card or bracelet with you.

Any unexplained malaise or fever should be promptly reported to your doctor, who will recommend bed rest and prescribe the appropriate kind of antibiotics for you. (Don't just self-treat the fever with any antibiotics you may have on hand; they may be inappropriate for the infection you have and may delay proper treatment by masking the problem.)

Cyanosis. This term refers to low oxygen levels in the blood, which causes a bluish discoloration of the skin. If you experience cyanosis, you will need special care to cope with polycythemia (a higher-than-normal red blood cell count), bleeding, and kidney problems. You will also need special counseling regarding pregnancy.

Contraception

If you have congenital heart disease and are considering a reliable form of contraception, you have a number of good choices available to you, the most reliable of which are oral contraceptives. Are oral contraceptives safe for women with congenital heart disease? The answer is usually yes. The only exceptions are if you have hypertension, pulmonary vascular disease, or cyanosis accompanied by an increased red blood cell count.

If you can't or don't want to use oral contraceptives, barrier methods (condom, diaphragm, contraceptive sponge, etc.) are safe and highly effective *when used as directed*. But barrier methods are not as effective as birth control pills.

The use of an intrauterine device (IUD) should probably be avoided, as it may increase the risk of bacterial endocarditis.

If you have a congenital heart defect in which pregnancy is not advised (such as pulmonary vascular disease or a right-to-left shunt, you should consider having a tubal ligation, in which the fallopian tubes leading from the ovaries to the uterus (and where conception normally takes place) are blocked with clips or rings or are surgically severed. Tubal ligation provides virtually foolproof permanent contraception.

Pregnancy

If you have congenital heart disease and are now in your twenties or thirties and contemplating starting a family, you're in good company. The number of women with congenital heart defects who have reached childbearing age has risen dramatically over the past thirty years. By some estimates, around 10 percent of women with heart disease during pregnancy are those with congenital heart defects.

Women with certain kinds of congenital heart defects tolerate pregnancy well. These include women with a left-to-right shunt, those with mild regurgitation of blood in the heart valves, and those who have no symptoms. Others, however, cannot tolerate the rigors of pregnancy well at all, and should avoid getting pregnant altogether. At particularly high risk are women with a right-to-left shunt (known as Eisenmenger's Syndrome) and those with primary pulmonary hypertension (high blood pressure in the pulmonary artery leading from the lungs back to the heart). If you have a congenital heart defect that causes such symptoms as cyanosis, breathlessness, or arrhythmias, you should avoid pregnancy too.

You should be aware that if you have a congenital heart defect, the risk that your children will be born with congenital defects is greater than that of women with normally functioning hearts. You may want to discuss the risk—and what can be done about it—with a genetic counselor *before* you conceive.

Epilogue

THERE'S NO CURE for coronary artery disease, hypertension, stroke, and other common forms of cardiovascular disease—at least not yet. Fortunately, most of these forms of heart disease can be prevented. This means adopting a heart-healthy lifestyle early on—preferably before the increased heart disease risks associated with menopause kick in.

A low-fat, low-cholesterol, low-sodium diet and regular exercise are cornerstones to a program of heart disease prevention. If you smoke, quitting may be one of the kindest things you can do for your heart. And while alcohol is thought to provide some protection against coronary artery disease, too much alcohol can actually increase your risk of other forms of cardiovascular disease. So limit your consumption of alcohol.

You will also need to make regular visits to your physician, who can monitor your lipid levels to determine how effective your efforts are. Your doctor can also diagnose and help you control hypertension and diabetes, two other risk factors for heart disease. If additional measures are needed, such as cholesterol-lowering medications, postmenopausal estrogens, or even over-the-counter aspirin, your physician can provide advice and a prescription.

Resources and Support

For more information on heart disease and reducing your risk, contact the following organizations.

Cardiovascular Disease

American Heart Association
National Center
7320 Greenville Avenue
Dallas, TX 75231
(800) 242-8721

The AHA has a wealth of materials, including fact sheets, brochures, and audiovisuals, on cardiovascular disease and its prevention. Publications include: *What Every Woman Should Know about High Blood Pressure*; *About Your Heart and Blood Pressure*; *American Heart Association Diet: An Eating Plan for Healthy Americans*; *Exercise and Your Heart*, and more. Check your phone directory for a local chapter or contact the national office. Single copies of most publications are free.

National Heart, Lung, and Blood Institute (NHLBI)
Information Center
P.O. Box 30105
Bethesda, MD 20824-0105
(301) 951-3260

The NHLBI Information Center provides patient education materials on high blood pressure, cholesterol, cigarette smoking, obesity, and heart disease. Write or call to request a directory of publications.

Diabetes

American Diabetes Association
National Service Center
1660 Duke Street
Alexandria, VA 22314
(800) 232-3472

This voluntary health organization is dedicated to increasing public awareness of diabetes and promoting and supporting diabetes research. The ADA publishes exchange lists for meal planning, along with numerous other pamphlets, booklets, and books, most of which are available for a nominal fee. The ADA also compiles an annual *Buyer's Guide to Diabetes Products* and publishes *Diabetes Forecast*, a monthly magazine full of helpful information and tips for people with diabetes and their families. Look in the phone book for a local affiliate of the ADA, or write or call the national office for more information and a publication list.

National Diabetes Information Clearinghouse (NDIC)
One Information Way
Bethesda, MD 20892-3560

The NDIC, an information and referral service funded by the National Institutes of Health, provides pamphlets and booklets on diabetes care for patients and their families free or for a nominal fee. The clearinghouse maintains a current list of cookbooks for people with diabetes, as well as lists of publications on foot care, pregnancy, kidney disease, and more. Write or call with your queries or to request a complete publication list.

Nutrition and Weight Control

American Dietetic Association (ADA)
National Center for Nutrition and Dietetics
216 West Jackson Boulevard, Suite 800
Chicago, IL 60606–6995
(800) 366–1655 (9 A.M. to 4 P.M. Central Time)

The ADA offers cookbooks and other materials designed to educate consumers about food and nutrition. The National Center for Nutrition and Dietetics is a public education initiative of the ADA. The ADA's consumer nutrition hotline provides recorded messages on current issues in nutrition or the opportunity to speak with a registered dietitian. The ADA can also help you find a registered dietitian in your area.

U.S. Food and Drug Administration (FDA)
Office of Consumer Affairs, HFE-88
5600 Fishers Lane
Rockville, MD 20857
(301) 443–3170

The FDA provides publications on a wide range of topics, including general drug information, medical devices, and food and nutrition. The FDA also publishes a monthly publication, *FDA Consumer*, which reports on recent developments in the regulation of foods, drugs, and cosmetics. Recent issues have included articles on women and heart disease, heart bypass surgery, balloon angioplasty, dieting, nutrition for women, and tips on using the new food labels. A one-year subscription (10 issues) costs $15. To subscribe, contact the Superintendent of Documents, P.O. Box 371954, Pittsburgh, PA 15250–7954. To order materials, contact the FDA at the address above or contact the FDA consumer affairs office nearest you. Most materials are available free of charge.

Food and Nutrition Information Center (FNIC)
National Agricultural Library
10310 Baltimore Avenue, Room 304
Beltsville, MD 20705–2351
(301) 504–5917

The FNIC answers questions about food and nutrition and provides database searches, bibliographies, and resource guides on a variety of food and nutrition topics.

Taking Off Pounds Sensibly (TOPS) Club
4575 South Fifth Street
P.O. Box 07360
Milwaukee, WI 53207
(414) 482–4620

This organization provides group therapy for people who want to lose weight. Members are required to use physician-approved individual eating plans and physician-set weight-loss goals. Check your phone directory for a local chapter or write to the national office.

Overeaters Anonymous
P.O. Box 92870
Los Angeles, CA 90009

This support group for compulsive overeaters is based on the twelve-step program of Alcoholics Anonymous. Check the phone book for local groups.

Weight Watchers International
Jericho Atrium
500 North Broadway
Jericho, NY 11753–2196
(516) 939–0400

This organization hosts group meetings that offer a nutritionally sound weight-loss program as well as plenty of emotional support. Look in the phone book for a local affiliate or contact Weight Watchers International for more information.

Tobacco, Alcohol, and Substance Abuse

National Clearinghouse for Alcohol and Drug Abuse Information (NCADI)
P.O. Box 2345
Rockville, MD 20852
(800) 729–6686; (301) 468–2600

The NCADI provides print and audiovisual information about alcohol and other drugs. Publications for women include *Alcohol Alert #10*; *Alcohol, Tobacco and Other Drugs May Harm the Unborn*; and *Women and Alcohol*. Write or call for a publications list.

American Lung Association
1740 Broadway
New York, NY 10019
(212) 315–8700

The ALA and its local affiliates conduct smoking-cessation programs and offer a catalog of publications, including many on smoking. Contact your local ALA affiliate or write to the national office.

Women's Health

Women to Woman America
222 SW 36th Terrace
Gainesville, FL 32607

Women to Woman America is the educational initiative of the National Menopause Foundation, Inc., established to give voice to women asking questions about menopause and other midlife issues. A $50 membership includes an annual subscription to the *Women's Health Digest*, a quarterly medical journal for lay women, written by medical experts in simple language.

Glossary

Androgens: The hormones responsible for the development and maintenance of male sexual characteristics and reproductive function in men. Androgens are produced by the testes and adrenal glands in men, and in small amounts by the adrenal glands and the ovaries in women. Androgens are believed to raise LDL cholesterol and lower HDL cholesterol, thus possibly contributing to an increased risk of heart disease.

Angiotension-Converting Enzyme (ACE) Inhibitors: These drugs are potent dilators of the arteries and veins, and are generally prescribed to lower blood pressure.

Angina pectoris: A discomfort in the chest caused by reduced blood flow to the heart. Angina is usually triggered by exercise, exposure to cold, or stress, and is relieved by rest and relaxation.

Angiography: An X-ray examination of the coronary blood vessels in which a fluid is injected into the bloodstream and X rays are taken as the fluid passes through the coronary arteries.

Anticoagulants: (1) Substances produced by the artery walls that help to prevent the formation of blood clots or that help to break up existing blood clots. (2) Drugs, such as heparin and warfarin, given to help prevent the formation of blood clots in susceptible people.

Antioxidants: Substances that, in the body, bind to and neutralize highly charged particles known as oxygen free radicals. Oxygen free radicals cause oxidation of LDL cholesterol, which, in turn, is more likely to be deposited on artery walls than normal LDL cholesterol. Vitamins A, E, C, beta-carotene, and the trace mineral selenium are antioxidants. (*See also* Oxygen free radicals.)

Antiplatelets: Drugs that decrease the stickiness of platelets, thus helping to prevent the formation of blood clots. Aspirin is the most widely used antiplatelet drug. These drugs sometimes are referred to as platelet inhibitors.

Apolipoprotein: The protein part of lipoproteins that is responsible for transporting fat and cholesterol through the body. (*See also* Lipoprotein.)

Arrhythmias: Irregularities in the heart's rate or rhythms. There are several kinds of arrhythmias: **tachycardia** refers to a rapid heart beat above ninety to one hundred beats per minute. **Bradycardia** is an abnormally slow heart rate. **Atrial fibrillation** occurs when the heart's upper chambers begin to beat rapidly and irregularly, and **ventricular fibrillation** refers to rapid and irregular beating of the lower chambers of the heart. Ventricular fibrillation is a life-threatening medical emergency. **Heart block** is another type of arrhythmia characterized by a slowdown in the passage of electrical currents through the heart.

Atherosclerosis: Progressive narrowing of the coronary arteries due to the buildup of hard plaques, consisting of cholesterol, fat, calcium deposits, and other debris, along the inner walls of the arteries.

Atrial natriuretic factor (ANF): A hormone that appears to help blood-clotting substances (platelets) aggregate faster, promoting the development of blood clots. Many people with high blood pressure have elevated levels of ANF, which may help explain why they're at greater risk of suffering a heart attack or stroke.

Balloon angioplasty: A procedure in which a small balloon is inserted through a catheter into a coronary artery and inflated to unblock the artery. The procedure is also known as percutaneous transluminal coronary angioplasty, or PTCA.

Beta-blockers: Drugs that slow the heart rate and decrease the contracting power of the heart muscle. Beta-blockers are typically prescribed for the treatment of hypertension and angina.

Bile acids: These acids are made by the liver and take up residence in the small intestine, where their job is to help in the digestion and absorption of dietary fat and cholesterol.

Bile acid sequestrants: A class of drugs used to lower blood lipid levels. The drugs prevent bile acids in the intestines from circulating in the bloodstream. As a result, the liver makes more bile acids from cholesterol stores in the liver. As the liver's cholesterol reserves are reduced, LDL receptors in the liver become more active, taking LDL cholesterol from the bloodstream.

Blood pressure: The force exerted by blood on the artery walls as the heart beats. A blood pressure measurement consists of two numbers: the top number, or systolic pressure, is the force of blood against the artery walls as the heart contracts; the bottom number, or diastolic pressure, reflects blood pressure on the artery walls between heartbeats.

Calcium channel blockers: A class of drugs that dilate the coronary arteries by blocking the entry of calcium into the smooth muscle tissues of the heart and arteries. Calcium channel blockers are prescribed to help control angina and to treat other heart conditions, such as arrhythmias and hypertension.

Cardiac catheterization: A procedure used for diagnosing coronary artery disease and other heart problems in which one or more catheters (long, flexible tubes) are inserted into an artery or vein (usually in the groin) and guided into the heart, where they may be used to take blood pressure readings, collect blood samples, or inject a dye into the heart's chambers and coronary arteries.

Cardiopulmonary resuscitation (CPR): An emergency procedure, consisting of external heart massage and artificial respiration, used to revive a person who has collapsed, has no pulse, and has stopped breathing. The procedure is intended to restore blood circulation and prevent brain damage or death due to lack of oxygen.

Cardiovascular disease: Any of a number of illnesses affecting the heart and blood vessels, including coronary heart disease, high blood pressure, and stroke.

Cerebral hemorrhage: A type of stroke that occurs when a blood vessel in the brain breaks and causes excessive bleeding.

Cerebral embolism: A type of stroke in which a blood clot circulating in the bloodstream lodges in an artery leading to or in the brain, disrupting blood flow.

Cerebral thrombosis: A type of stroke in which a blood clot forms in an artery supplying blood to part of the brain and disrupts blood flow.

Cholesterol: A complex chemical found in all animal fats and in every cell in your body. Cholesterol plays a key role in the formation of cell membranes, and also helps in the manufacture of certain hormones. There are several kinds of cholesterol in the body, including low-density lipoprotein (LDL) cholesterol, believed to contribute to the development of heart disease, and high-density lipoprotein (HDL) cholesterol, believed to protect against heart disease by clearing LDL cholesterol from the bloodstream.

Cholestyramine: One of two types of bile acid sequestrants used to lower blood lipid levels. (*See also* Bile acid sequestrants.)

Coagulants: Substances in the bloodstream, produced by the blood vessel walls that are instrumental in the development of blood clots.

Colestipol: One of two types of bile acid sequestrants used to lower blood lipids. (*See also* Bile acid sequestrants.)

Coronary artery disease: A form of cardiovascular disease that occurs when deposits of fat, calcium, and scar tissue gradually build up on the inner walls of the coronary arteries, the blood vessels that supply nutrients and oxygen to the heart muscle. The deposits result in reduced or complete blockages of blood flow to the heart.

Coronary thrombosis: A blood clot that forms in the coronary arteries, usually resulting in a heart attack.

Diabetes mellitus: Abnormally high blood sugar levels caused when the body either doesn't produce enough insulin or is unable to use insulin efficiently. There are two forms. Type I (juvenile-onset) diabetes usually develops before age twenty-five. These people produce very little insulin and must take insulin injections to control blood sugar levels. Type II, or adult-onset, diabetes typically develops in adulthood (after age forty). In many Type II diabetics, the pancreas produces insulin, but the body somehow becomes resistant to insulin's effects on blood sugar. Type II diabetes can often be controlled through dietary and weight-loss measures.

Diastolic blood pressure: *See* Blood pressure.

Dietary fiber: The indigestible part of plant foods. There are two types: (1) water-insoluble fiber, which doesn't dissolve in water and is found mostly in wheat bran and whole wheat products; and (2) water-soluble fiber, which dissolves in water and forms a gummy gel. Foods high in soluble fiber include oat bran, fruits and vegetables, and dried peas and beans.

Echocardiography: A diagnostic test in which high-frequency sound waves (ultrasound) are used to view the physical anatomy and structure of the heart.

Electrocardiogram (ECG): A diagnostic test that measures the heart rate and its electrical activity.

Endothelium: The inner lining of the artery.

Estrogen: A female sex hormone produced by the ovaries that helps regulate a woman's monthly menstrual cycle. Estrogen is believed to help protect women from heart disease in their childbearing years. Postmenopausal estrogen preparations have been found to extend that protection after menopause.

Exercise stress test: An electrocardiogram that measures your heart rate and its electrical activity as you exercise on a treadmill or stationary bicycle. The test is used to detect such heart problems as angina or ischemia (reduced blood flow to the heart). It is also useful in determining your level of physical fitness before launching an exercise program.

Fasting blood glucose test: A screening test for diabetes in which blood glucose levels are measured after a twelve-hour fast.

Ferritin: A protein circulating in the bloodstream that reflects the amount of iron stored in body tissues. Some studies have suggested that high ferritin levels may be associated with an increased risk of heart disease.

Fibric acids: Drugs used to reduce the risk of pancreatitis (inflammation of the pancreas) among people with high blood triglycerides. Gemfibrozil, the more widely used, has also been found to protect against heart disease.

Fibrinogen: A blood coagulant that helps form blood clots. High blood levels of fibrinogen have been associated with an increased risk of heart disease.

Foam cells: White blood cells residing in the artery wall that have become saturated with cholesterol. Foam cells are believed to be precursors to artery-clogging plaques.

Heart attack: A condition in which one or more of the coronary arteries that supply the heart muscle with nutrients and oxygen become blocked, either by progressive narrowing (stenosis) or by a blood clot (thrombosis). With no oxygen and nutrients, the heart tissue supplied by the blocked artery begins to die.

Hemostasis: The body's system of controlling blood flow and blood clotting.

High-density lipoprotein (HDL) cholesterol: The "good" cholesterol believed to protect against heart disease by clearing LDL cholesterol from the bloodstream.

HMG CoA reductase inhibitors: A class of drugs that lower blood lipids by inhibiting the enzyme HMG CoA reductase, which regulates the amount of cholesterol manufactured by the liver. These include lovastatin (Mevacor), simvastatin (Zocor), and pravastatin (Pravachol).

Hypertension: A condition in which a person's blood pressure is higher than normal. People with two or more blood pressure readings over 140/90 are considered to have hypertension and to be at a greater risk of having a heart attack, stroke, or kidney disease. (*See also* Blood pressure.)

Insulin: A hormone secreted by the pancreas. Insulin helps maintain blood sugar levels. Insulin is also believed to be instrumental in the development of heart disease by stimulating the sympathetic nervous system, and causing the kidneys to retain sodium, both of which can raise blood pressure. Insulin may also damage the lining of the artery, encouraging the development of plaques. (*See also* Diabetes mellitus.)

Left ventricular hypertrophy: A condition associated with prolonged hypertension in which the heart wall thickens. As a result, the heart pumps blood less efficiently. Left ventricular hypertrophy can lead to congestive heart failure.

Lipid profile: A blood test used to determine levels of total cholesterol, low-density lipoproteins (LDL cholesterol), high-density lipoproteins (HDL cholesterol), triglycerides, and the ratio of total cholesterol to HDL cholesterol. Test results are used to help assess a person's risk of developing heart disease.

Lipids: A variety of fats that circulate in the bloodstream, including triglycerides, very-low-density lipoproteins, low-density lipoproteins, and high-density lipoproteins.

Lipoproteins: Fat and cholesterol that have been packaged along with protein carriers (called apolipoproteins) by the liver, thus allowing the fats to circulate in the bloodstream. There are several types of lipoproteins: very-low-density lipoproteins (VLDL), low-density lipoproteins (LDL), and high-density lipoproteins (HDL).

Lipoprotein (a): One of numerous protein carriers, or apolipoproteins, that transports fat and cholesterol through the bloodstream. High blood levels of lipoprotein (a) have been associated with a strong risk of heart attack.

Low-density lipoprotein (LDL) cholesterol: The "bad" cholesterol believed to contribute to coronary artery disease by accumulating on the artery walls, forming hard plaques that reduce blood flow.

Macrophages: White blood cells that rove through the body, attacking foreign invaders. When macrophages take up residence in the artery wall, they attract and absorb fat, forming foam cells, the precursors of plaques.

Menopause: The final menstrual period that marks the end of a woman's childbearing years, usually occurring around age fifty. After menopause, levels of the reproductive hormone estrogen decline.

Microvascular angina: Chest pain that occurs when the coronary arteries go into spasm, temporarily reducing blood flow to the heart muscle. Usually diagnostic tests reveal no evidence of blockage of the arteries. The condition often responds well to treatment with estrogen.

Mitral valve prolapse: A condition in which one or both leaflets that make up the mitral valve of the heart billow up into the heart's atrial chamber, often resulting in a clicking sound or heart murmur. The condition, while usually harmless, can cause bothersome symptoms, including heart palpitations and chest pain.

Monounsaturated fats: *See* Unsaturated fat.

Myocardial infarction: The medical term for heart attack. (*See also* Heart attack.)

Niacin (Nicotinic acid): A B vitamin primarily found in milk, eggs, fish, and poultry. A prescription form of niacin is used to lower blood cholesterol.

Nitrates: Drugs that dilate the coronary arteries and are often prescribed to treat angina pectoris. Also known as nitroglycerine.

Omega-3 fatty acids: A type of polyunsaturated fat that's found mostly in fish and is believed to protect against heart disease by reducing the stickiness of platelets.

Orthostatic hypotension: A drop in blood pressure that occurs when blood pools in the legs while a person is seated or lying down and doesn't rise quickly enough to supply the brain with sufficient blood or oxygen when the person stands up. The condition, sometimes referred to as postural hypotension, may cause dizziness and, in severe cases, fainting.

Oxygen free radicals: Highly charged particles that are missing one electron, occurring naturally in the environment and in the body as a byproduct of metabolism. These unstable molecules literally bombard other cells in the body in an attempt to pair up with another electron. The force of the collision can damage cell membranes, a process known as oxidation. Oxidation of LDL cholesterol may be partly responsible for the formation of atherosclerotic plaques on the artery walls. Antioxidants can help prevent oxidation.

Percutaneous transluminal coronary angioplasty: *See* Balloon angioplasty.

Plaque: A buildup of cholesterol, calcium deposits, scar tissue, and other debris on the inner linings of the arteries.

Platelets: Substances that help blood coagulate and form clots.

Polyunsaturated fats: *See* Unsaturated fat.

Probucol: A drug that moderately lowers LDL cholesterol.

Progesterone: A female sex hormone produced by the ovaries that helps thicken the lining of the uterus each month in preparation for pregnancy.

Progestogen: A synthetic form of progesterone used in birth control pills and postmenopausal hormone therapy.

Prostacyclin: A substance secreted by the blood vessel wall that helps prevent platelets from sticking together and dilates the blood vessel, improving blood flow.

Psyllium: A type of soluble fiber found in bulk fiber laxatives and in some breakfast cereals. Psyllium has been found to lower cholesterol.

Saturated fat: A type of fatty acid that's "saturated" with hydrogen atoms. These fats, found in butter, whole milk, ice cream, eggs, red meat and other animal foods, are solid at room temperature. A diet high in saturated fats is associated with high blood cholesterol levels.

Sodium: A metallic element that, in the body, is responsible for acid-base balance, water balance, nerve transmission, and muscle contraction. Sodium is also a main component of ordinary table salt.

Soluble fiber: *See* Dietary fiber.

Stroke: A disruption of blood flow to the brain caused by excessive bleeding (hemorrhagic stroke) or by a blood clot.

Subarachnoid hemorrhage: A type of stroke that occurs when a blood vessel on the surface of the brain ruptures and bleeds into the space between the brain and the skull.

Surgical menopause: An abrupt cessation of menstruation brought on by the sudden severing of estrogen and progesterone after surgical removal of the ovaries.

Sympathetic nervous system: Part of the autonomic nervous system that involves such involuntary reflexes as breathing and heart rate.

Systolic blood pressure: *See* Blood pressure.

Thallium exercise stress test: A diagnostic test to detect blockages in the coronary arteries. The test is identical to the exercise stress test with one exception: at the peak of exercise, or immediately afterward, a small amount of radioactive thallium is injected into a vein in your arm. The amount of radioactive gamma rays detected by a hand-held gamma counter immediately after the test and again several hours later helps determine the extent of the blockage.

Thiazide diuretics: One of the most commonly prescribed antihypertensive medications. These drugs work on the kidneys and rid the body of sodium while retaining calcium.

Thrombolytic drugs: Drugs used to break up blood clots following a heart attack or stroke.

Trans fatty acids: Fatty acids in margarines and spreads created when unsaturated fats are hydrogenated, or hardened. Trans fatty acids have been found to raise blood cholesterol levels, and diets high in trans fatty acids have been associated with an increased risk of heart disease.

Transient ischemic attack (TIA): A condition in which blood flow to part of the brain is temporarily disrupted by spasm or a blood clot, triggering such symptoms as temporary weakness, clumsiness, or loss of feeling in an arm, leg, or side of the face. TIAs are a warning sign of stroke.

Triglycerides: A type of fat that circulates in the bloodstream, and is either used for energy or stored in the body's tissues as fat. Triglycerides can be manufactured by the liver and also come from dietary fat.

Unsaturated fats: Fats that are liquid at room temperature, including safflower oil, sunflower oil, and corn oil. Unsaturated fats are known to help lower blood cholesterol levels.

Selected Bibliography

Introduction

Barnard, R. J. "Effects of Life-Style Modification on Serum Lipids." *Archives of Internal Medicine*. 1991; 151:1389–1394.

Healy, B. "The Yentl Syndrome." *New England Journal of Medicine*. 1991; 325:274–276.

Heart and Stroke Facts: 1994 Statistical Supplement. 1994, American Heart Association.

Heart Disease in African-American Women. 1994, American Heart Association.

Rich-Edwards, J. W., J. E. Manson, C. H. Hennekens, and J. E. Buring. "The Primary Prevention of Coronary Heart Disease in Women." *New England Journal of Medicine*. 1995; 332:1759–1766.

Johnson, C. L., B. M. Rifkind, C. T. Sempos, et al. "Declining Serum Total Cholesterol Levels among US Adults: The National Health and Nutrition Examination Surveys." *Journal of the American Medical Association*. 1993; 269(23):3002–3008.

Leaf, A., and T. J. Ryan. "Prevention of Coronary Artery Disease: A Medical Imperative" (Editorial). *New England Journal of Medicine*. 1990; 323(20):1416–1419.

Lerner, D. J. and W. B. Kannel. "Patterns of Coronary Heart Disease Morbidity and Mortality in the Sexes: A 26-Year Follow-up of the Framingham Population." 1986; 111:383.

Manson, J. E., H. Tosteson, P. M. Ridker, et al. "The Primary Prevention of Myocardial Infarction." *New England Journal of Medicine*. 1992; 326(21):1406–1416.

Ornish, D., S. E. Brown, L. W. Scherwitz, et al. "Can Lifestyle Changes

Reverse Coronary Heart Disease? The Lifestyle Heart Trial." *Lancet.* 1990; 336:129–33.

Stehbens, W. E. "An Appraisal of the Epidemic Rise of Coronary Heart Disease and Its Decline." *Lancet.* 1987; 606–610

Tobin, N. J., S. Wassertheil-Smoller, J. P. Wexler, et al. "Sex Bias in Considering Coronary Bypass Surgery." *Annals of Internal Medicine.* 1987; 107:19–25.

Walter, H. J., A. Hofman, R. D. Vaughan, and E. L. Wydner. "Modification of Risk Factors for Coronary Heart Disease: Five-Year Results of a School-Based Intervention Trial." *New England Journal of Medicine.* 1988; 318:1093–1100.

Wenger, N. K., L. Speroff, and B. Packard. "Cardiovascular Health and Disease in Women." *New England Journal of Medicine.* 1993; 329(4):247–256.

Chapter 1: The Healthy Heart

Cannon, R. O. "Chest Pain with Normal Coronary Angiograms" (Editorial). *New England Journal of Medicine.* 1993; 328(23):1706–1708.

Egashira, K., T. Inou, Y. Hirooka, et al. "Evidence of Impaired Endothelium-Dependent Coronary Vasodilation in Patients with Angina Pectoris and Normal Coronary Angiograms." *New England Journal of Medicine.* 1993; 328–1659–1664.

Luscher, T. F. "The Endothelium and Cardiovascular Disease—A Complex Relation." *New England Journal of Medicine.* 1994; 330(15):1081–1083.

Sarrel, P. M., D. Lindsay, G. M. C. Rosano, and P. A. Poole-Wilson. "Angina and Normal Coronary Arteries in Women: Gynecological Findings." *American Journal of Obstetrics and Gynecology.* 1992; 167:467–472.

Tofler, G. H., P. H. Stone, J. E. Muller, et al. "Clinical Manifestations of Coronary Heart Disease in Women." In Eaker E. D., B. Packard, N. J. Wenger, et al. (eds.). *Coronary Heart Disease in Women.* New York: Haymarket Doyma, 1987.

Chapter 2: How Men and Women Are Different

Fields, S. K., M. A. Savard, and K. R. Epstein. "The Female Patient." In Douglas, P. S. (ed.), *Cardiovascular Health and Disease in Women.* Philadelphia: W. B. Saunders Company, 1992.

Ness, R. A., T. Harris, J. Cobb, et al. "Number of Pregnancies and the Subsequent Risk of Cardiovascular Disease." *New England Journal of Medicine.* 1993; 328:1528–1533.

Chapter 3: How Coronary Artery Disease Develops

Allemann, Y. F. F. Horber, M. Colombo, P. Ferrari, S. Shaw, P. Jaeger, and P. Weidmann. "Insulin Sensitivity and Body Fat Distribution in Normotensive Offspring of Hypertensive Parents." *Lancet*. 1993; 341:327–331.

"Atherosclerosis Goes to the Wall" (Editorial). *Lancet*. 1992; 339:647–648.

Austin, M. A., J. N. Breslow, C. H. Hennekens, et al. "Low-Density Lipoprotein Subclass Patterns and Risk of Myocardial Infarction." *Journal of the American Medical Association*. 1988; 260:1917–1921.

Bergqvist, A. D. Bergqvist, and M. Fernö. "Estrogen and Progesterone Receptors in Vessel Walls: Biochemical and Immunological Assays." *Acta Obstet Gynecol Scand*. 1993; 72:10–16.

de Graff, J., H. L. M. Hak-Lemmers, M. P. C. Hectors, et al. "Enhanced Susceptibility to In Vitro Oxidation of the Dense Low-Density Lipoprotein Subfractions in Healthy Subjects." *Arteriosclerosis*. 1991; 11:298–306.

Eckel, R. H. "Insulin Resistance: An Adaptation for Weight Maintenance." *Lancet*. 1992; 340:1452–1453.

Fuster, V., L. Badimon, J. J. Badimon, and J. H. Chesebro. "The Pathogenesis of Coronary Artery Disease and the Acute Coronary Syndromes." In Epstein, F. H. (ed). "Mechanisms of Disease." *New England Journal of Medicine*. 1992; 326(4):242–250.

Galli, S. J. "New Concepts About the Mast Cell." In Flier, J. S., and L. H. Underhill (eds.). "Seminars in Medicine of the Beth Israel Hospital, Boston." *New England Journal of Medicine*. 1993; 328(4):257–265.

Hamsten, A. "Hemostatic Function and Coronary Artery Disease" (Editorial). *New England Journal of Medicine*. 1995; 332:677–678.

Hansson, G. K. "Atherosclerosis: Immunological Markers of Atherosclerosis" (Commentary). *Lancet*. 1993; 341:278.

"Hypertriglyceridaemia and Vascular Risk." Report of a Meeting of Physicians and Scientists, University College London Medical School. *Lancet*. 1993; 342:781–786.

Johnston, R. B., Jr. "Current Concepts: Immunology, Monocytes and Macrophages." *New England Journal of Medicine*. 1988; 318(12):747–752.

Lobo, R. A., M. Notelovitz, L. Bernstein, F. Y. Khan, R. K. Ross, and W. L. Paul. "Lp(a) Lipoprotein: Relationship to Cardiovascular Disease Risk Factors, Exercise, and Estrogen." *American Journal of Obstetrics and Gynecology*. 1992; 166(4):1182–1190.

"Low Cholesterol and Increased Risk." *Lancet*. 1989; 1423–1425.

Qingbo, X. J. Willeit, M. Marosi, et al. "Association of Serum Antibodies to Heat-Shock Protein 65 with Carotid Atherosclerosis." *Lancet*. 1993; 341(8840):255–259.

Remuzzi, G. and A. Benigni. "Endothelins in the Control of Cardiovascular and Renal Function." *Lancet.* 1993; 342:589–593.

Ridker, P. M., D. E. Vaughan, and M. J. Stampfer. "Endogenous Tissue-Type Plasminogen Activator and Risk of Myocardial Infarction." *Lancet.* 1993; 341(8854):1166–1168.

Seed, M. F. Hoppichler, D. Reaveley,? McCarthy, et al. "Relation of Serum Lipoprotein(a) Concentration and Apolipoprotein(a) Phenotype to Coronary Heart Disease in Patients with Familial Hypercholesterolemia." *New England Journal of Medicine.* 1990; 322(21):1494–1498.

Stout, R. W. "Insulin and Atheroma—An Update" *Lancet.* 1987; 1077–1079.

Thompson, S. G., J. Kienast, S. D. M. Pyke, F. Haverkate, and J. C. W. van de Loo. "Hemostatic Factors and the Risk of Myocardial Infarction or Sudden Death in Patients with Angina Pectoris." *New England Journal of Medicine.* 1995; 332:635–641.

Ware, A. W. and D. D. Heistad. "Platelet-Endothelium Interactions." In Flier, J. S., and L. H. Underhill (eds.). "Seminars in Medicine of the Beth Israel Hospital, Boston." *New England Journal of Medicine.* 1993; 328(9):628–635.

Chapter 4: Are You at Risk?

Anderson, H. V., and J. T. Willerson. "Thrombolysis in Acute Myocardial Infarction." *New England Journal of Medicine.* 1993; 329(10):703–709.

Barrett-Connor, E. L., B. A. Cohn, D. L. Wingard, and S. L. Edelstein. "Why Is Diabetes Mellitus a Stronger Risk Factor for Fatal Ischemic Heart Disease in Women Than in Men? The Rancho Bernardo Study." *Journal of the American Medical Association.* 1991; 265(5):627–631.

Bush, T. L. "The Epidemiology of Cardiovascular Disease in Postmenopausal Women." *Annals of the New York Academy of Science.* 1990; 592:263–271.

Castelli, W. P. "The Triglyceride Issue: A View from Framingham." *American Heart Journal.* 1986; 112: 432–437.

den Heijer, M., H. J. Blom, W. B. J. Gerrits, F. R. Rosendaal, H. L. Haak, P. W. Wijermans, and G. M. J. Bos. "Is Hyperhomocysteinaemia a Risk Factor for Recurrent Venous Thrombosis?" *Lancet.* 1995; 345:882–885.

Glantz, S. A., and W. W. Parmley. "Passive Smoking and Heart Disease." *Journal of the American Medical Association.* 1995; 273:1047–1053.

Keil, J. E., S. E. Sutherland, R. G. Knapp, et al. "Mortality Rates and Risk Factors for Coronary Disease in Black as Compared with White Men and Women." *New England Journal of Medicine.* 1993; 329(2):73–78.

Lesko, S. M., L. Rosenberg, and S. Shapiro. "A Case-Control Study of Baldness in Relation to Myocardial Infarction in Men." *Journal of the American Medical Association.* 1993; 269(8):998–1003.

Mahley, R. W., K. H. Weisgraber, T. L. Innerarity, and S. C. Rall. "Genetic

Defects in Lipoprotein Metabolism." *Journal of the American Medical Association.* 1991; 265(1):78–83.

Manson, J. E., G. A. Colditz, M. J. Stampfer, et al. "A Prospective Study of Obesity and Risk of Coronary Heart Disease in Women." *New England Journal of Medicine.* 1990; 332:882–889.

Manson, J. E., M. J. Stampfer, C. H. Hennekens, and W. C. Willet. "Body Weight and Longevity: A Reassessment." *Journal of the American Medical Association.* 1987; 257(3):353–358.

Matthews, K. A., E. Meilahn, L. H. Kuller, et al. "Menopause and Risk Factors for Coronary Heart Disease." *New England Journal of Medicine.* 1989; 321:641–646.

NIH Consensus Development Panel on Triglyceride, High-Density Lipoprotein, and Coronary Heart Disease. "Triglyceride, High-Density Lipoprotein, and Coronary Heart Disease." *Journal of the American Medical Association.* 1993; 269:505–510.

Ostlund, R. E., M. Staten, W. M. Kohrt, et al. "The Ratio of Waist-to-Hip Circumference, Plasma Insulin Level, and Glucose Intolerance as Independent Predictors of the HDL2 Cholesterol Level in Older Adults." *New England Journal of Medicine.* 1990; 322:229–234.

Remuzzi, G., and A Benigni. "Endothelins in the Control of Cardiovascular and Renal Function." *Lancet.* 1993; 342:589–593.

Stampfer, M. J., and M. R. Malinow. "Can Lowering Homocysteine Levels Reduce Cardiovascular Risk?" (Editorial). *New England Journal of Medicine.* 1995; 332:328–329.

Wei, J. Y. "Age and the Cardiovascular System." *New England Journal of Medicine.* 1992; 327(24):1735–1739.

Willett, W. C., J. E. Manson, M. J. Stampfer, et al. "Weight, Weight Change and Coronary Heart Disease in Women: Risk Within the 'Normal' Weight Range." *Journal of the American Medical Association.* 1995; 273(6):461–465.

Wilson, P. W. F., and W. B. Kannel. "Is Baldness Bad for the Heart?" (Editorial). *Journal of the American Medical Association.* 1993; 269(8):1035–1036.

Wing, R. R., K. A. Matthews, L. H. Kuller, et al. "Environmental and Familial Contributions to Insulin Levels and Change in Insulin Levels in Middle-aged Women." *Journal of the American Medical Association.* 1992; 268(14):1890–1895.

Chapter 5: Common Screening and Diagnostic Tests

Expert Panel on Detection, Evaluation, and Treatment of High Blood Cholesterol in Adults. "Summary of the Second Report of the National Cholesterol Education Program (NCEP) Expert Panel on Detection, Evaluation, and

Treatment of High Blood Cholesterol in Adults (Adult Treatment Panel II)." *Journal of the American Medical Association*. 1993: 269(23):3015–3023.

Folsom, A. R., S. A. Kay, T. A. Sellers, et al. "Body Fat Distribution and 5-Year Risk of Death in Older Women." *Journal of the American Medical Association*. 1993; 269(4):483–487.

Gordon, D. J., J. L. Probstfield, R. F. Garrison, et al. "High-Density Lipoprotein Cholesterol and Cardiovascular Disease: Four Prospective Studies." *Circulation*. 1989; 79:8–15.

Hulley, S. B., T. B. Newman, D. Grady, et al. "Should We Be Measuring Blood Cholesterol Levels in Young Adults?" *Journal of the American Medical Association*. 1993; 269(11):1416–1419.

Murray, P. M., and J. D. Cantwell. "Prevalence of False-Positive Exercise Tests in Apparently Normal Women." *The Physician and Sportsmedicine*. 1988; 16(1):75–79.

Notelovitz, M., C. Fields, K. Caramelli, M. Dougherty, and A. L. Schwartz. "Cardiorespiratory Fitness Evaluation in Climacteric Women: Comparison of Two Methods." *American Journal of Obstetrics and Gynecology*. 1986; 154(5):1009–1013.

Sempos, C. T., J. I. Cleeman, M. D. Carroll, et al. "Prevalence of High Blood Cholesterol Among U.S. Adults." *Journal of the American Medical Association*. 1993; 269(23):3009–3014.

Chapter 6: A Prudent Diet for the Prevention of Coronary Artery Disease

Anderson, J. W., B. M. Smith, and N. J. Gustafson. "Health Benefits and Practical Aspects of High-Fiber Diets." *American Journal of Clinical Nutrition*. 1994:59(Suppl.) 1242S–1247S.

Brownell, K. D. "Differential Changes in Plasma High-Density Lipoprotein-Cholesterol Levels in Obese Men and Women During Weight Reduction." *Archives of Internal Medicine*. 1981; 141:1142–1146.

Danforth, E., and E. A. H. Sims. "Obesity and Efforts to Lose Weight" (Editorial). *New England Journal of Medicine*. 1992; 327:1947–1948.

Dreon, D. M., K. M. Vranizan, R. M. Krauss, M. A. Austin, and P. D. Wood. "The Effects of Polyunsaturated Fat vs. Monounsaturated Fat on Plasma Lipoproteins." *Journal of the American Medical Association*. 1990; 263:2462–2466.

Hankinson S. E., and M. J. Stampfer. "All That Glitters Is Not Beta-Carotene" (Editorial). *Journal of the American Medical Association*. 1994; 272(18):1455–1456.

Hennekens, C. H., J. E. Burning, and R. Peto. "Antioxidant Vitamins—

Benefits Not Yet Proved" (Editorial). *The New England Journal of Medicine.* 1994; 330:1080–1081.

Hertog, M. G. L., J. M. Feskens, P. C. H. Hollman, et al. "Dietary Antioxidant Flavonoids and Risk of Coronary Heart Disease: The Zutphen Elderly Study." *Lancet.* 1993; 342:1007–1011.

Hodis, H. N., W. J. Mack, L. LaBree, L. Cashin-Hemphill, A. Sevanian, R. Johnson, and S. P. Azen. "Serial Coronary Angiographic Evidence That Antioxidant Vitamin Intake Reduces Progress of Coronary Artery Athero-sclerosis." *Journal of the American Medical Association.* 1995; 273:1849–1854.

Hunninghake, D. B., E. A. Stein, C. A. Dujovne, et al. "Efficacy of Intensive Dietary Therapy Alone or Combined with Lovastatin in Outpatients with Hypercholesterolemia." *New England Journal of Medicine.* 1993; 328(17):1213–1225.

Katan, M. B. "Fish and Heart Disease" (Editorial). *New England Journal of Medicine.* 1995; 332:1024–1025.

Leaf, A., and P. C. Weber. "Cardiovascular Effects of n-3 Fatty Acids." *New England Journal of Medicine.* 1988; 318:549–557.

Lichtman, S. W., K. Pisarska, E. R. Berman, M. Pestone, H. Dowling, E. Offenbacher, H. Weisel, S. Heshka, D. E. Matthews, and S. B. Heymsfield. "Discrepancy Between Self-Reported and Actual Caloric Intake and Exercise in Obese Subjects." *New England Journal of Medicine.* 1992; 327:1893–1898.

Mann, G. V. "Metabolic Consequences of Dietary Trans Fatty Acids." *Lancet.* 1994; 343:1268–1271.

Morris, D. L., S. B. Kritchevsky, and C. E. Davis. "Serum Carotenoids and Coronary Heart Disease: The Lipid Research Clinics Coronary Primary Prevention Trial and Follow-up Study." *Journal of the American Medical Association.* 1994; 272(18):1439–1441.

Ornish, D., S. E. Brown, L. W. Scherwitz, et al. "Can Lifestyle Changes Reverse Coronary Heart Disease? The Lifestyle Heart Trial." *Lancet.* 1990; 336:129–133.

Sabate, J., G. E. Fraser, K. Burke, S. F. Knutsen, H. Bennett, and K. D. Lindsted. "Effects of Walnuts on Serum Lipid Levels and Blood Pressure in Normal Men." *New England Journal of Medicine.* 1993; 328:603–607.

Sempos, C. T., J. I. Cleeman, M. D. Carroll, et al. "Prevalence of High Blood Cholesterol Among U.S. Adults." *Journal of the American Medical Association.* 1993; 269(23):3009–3014.

Soo-Sang, K., P. W. K. Wong, H. Y. Cook, M. Norusis, and J. V. Messer. "Protein-Bound Homocyst(e)ine: A Possible Risk Factor for Coronary Artery Disease." *Journal of Clinical Investigation.* 1986; 77:1482–1486.

Stampfer, M. J., C. H. Hennekens, J. E Manson, et al. "Vitamin E Consump-tion and the Risk of Coronary Heart Disease in Women." *New England Journal of Medicine.* 1993; 328:1444–1449.

Steinberg, D. "Antioxidant Vitamins and Coronary Heart Disease" (Editorial). *New England Journal of Medicine*. 1993; 328(20):1487–1489.

Willett, W. C., and A. Scherio. "Trans Fatty Acids: Are the Effects Only Marginal?" *American Journal of Public Health*. 1994; 84:722–724.

Willett, W. C., M. J. Stampfer, J. E. Manson, et al. "Intake of Trans Fatty Acids and Risk of Coronary Heart Disease Among Women." *Lancet*. 1993; 341:581–585.

Chapter 7: Exercising Your Option for a Healthier Heart

Blackburn, H. and D. R. Jacobs. "Physical Activity and the Risk of Coronary Heart Disease" (Editorial). *New England Journal of Medicine*. 1988; 319:1217–1219.

Blair, S. N., H. W. Kohl, R. S. Paffenbarger, et al. "Physical Fitness and All-Cause Mortality: A Prospective Study of Healthy Men and Women." *Journal of the American Medical Association*. 1989; 262(17):2395–2401.

Blumenthal, J. A., K. Matthews, M. Fredrikson, N. Rifai, S. Schmiebolk, D. German, J. Steege, J. Rodin. "Effects of Exercise Training on Cardiovascular Function and Plasma Lipid, Lipoprotein, and Apolipoprotein Concentrations in Premenopausal and Postmenopausal Women." *Arteriosclerosis and Thrombosis*. 1991; 11:912–917.

Busby, J., M. Notelovitz, K. Putney, and T. Grow. "Exercise, High-Density Lipoprotein-Cholesterol, and Cardiorespiratory Function in Climacteric Women." *Southern Medical Journal*. 1985; 78:769–773.

"Coronary Heart Disease Attributable to Sedentary Lifestyle—Selected States, 1988." *Journal of the American Medical Association* 1990; 264(11):1390–1392.

Curfman, G. D. "The Health Benefits of Exercise" (Editorial). *New England Journal of Medicine*. 1993; 328:574–576.

Fletcher, G. F., S. N. Blair, J. Blumenthal, C. Caspersen, B. Chaitman, S. Epstein, H. Falls, E. S. S. Froelicher, V. F. Froelicher, and I. L. Pina. "AHA Medical/Scientific Statement: Position Statement on Exercise—Benefits and Recommendations for Physical Activity Programs for All Americans, A Statement for Health Professionals by the Committee on Exercise and Cardiac Rehabilitation of the Council on Clinical Cardiology, American Heart Association." *American Heart Association*. 1992.

Harris, S. S., C. J. Caspersen, G. H. DeFriese, and E. H. Estes, Jr. "Physical Activity Counseling for Healthy Adults as a Primary Preventive Intervention in the Clinical Setting." *Journal of the American Medical Association*. 1989; 261:3590–3598.

Horton, E. S. "Exercise and Decreased Risk of NIDDM" (Editorial). *New England Journal of Medicine*. 1991; 325:196–197.

Kelemen, M. H., M. B. Effron, S. A. Valenti, and K. J. Stewart. "Exercise Training Combined with Antihypertensive Drug Therapy—Effects on Lipids, Blood Pressure, and Left Ventricular Mass." *Journal of the American Medical Association.* 1990; 263:2766–2771.

Koplan, J. P., C. J. Caspersen, and K. E. Powell. "Physical Activity, Physical Fitness, and Health: Time to Act" (Editorial). *Journal of the American Medical Association.* 1989; 262:2437.

Martin, A. D., M. Notelovitz, C. Fields, and J. O'Kroy. "Predicting Maximal Oxygen Uptake from Treadmill Testing in Trained and Untrained Women." *American Journal of Obstetrics and Gynecology.* 1989; 161(5):1127–1132.

Muller, J. E., and G. H. Tofler. "Circadian Variation and Cardiovascular Disease" (Editorial). *New England Journal of Medicine.* 1991; 325:1038–1039.

Notelovitz, M. "Exercise, Nutrition, and the Coagulation Effects of Estrogen Replacement on Cardiovascular Health." *Obstetric and Gynecology Clinics of North America.* 1987; 14(1):121–141.

Pate, R. P., M. Pratt, S. N. Blair, et al. "Physical Activity and Public Health: A Recommendation from the Centers for Disease Control and Prevention and the American College of Sports Medicine." *Journal of the American Medical Association.* 1995; 273(5):402–407.

Probart, C. K., M. Notelovitz, D. Martin, F. Y. Khan, and C. Fields. "The Effect of Moderate Aerobic Exercise on Physical Fitness Among Women 70 Years and Older." *Maturitas.* 1991; 14:49–56.

Reaven, P. D., J. B McPhillips, E. L. Barrett-Connor, and M. H. Criqui. "Leisure Time Exercise and Lipid and Lipoprotein Levels in an Older Population." *Journal of the American Geriatric Society.* 1990; 38:847–854.

Ruys, T., M. Shaikh, B. G. Nordestgarrd, I. Sturgess, G. F. Watts, and B. Lewis. "Effect of Exercise and Fat Ingestion on High Density Lipoprotein production by Peripheral Tissues." *Lancet.* 1989; 1119–1122.

Van Dam, S., M. Gillespy, M. Notelovitz, and A. D. Martin. "Effect of Exercise on Glucose Metabolism in Postmenopausal Women." *American Journal of Obstetrics and Gynecology.* 1988; 159:82–86.

Zauner, C. W., M. Notelovitz, C. D. Fields, K. M. Clair, W. J. Clair, and R. B. Vogel. "Cardiorespiratory Efficiency at Submaximal Work in Young and Middle-aged Women" *American Journal of Obstetrics and Gynecology.* 1984; 150:712–715.

Chapter 8: Other Ways to Reduce Your Risk

Manson, J. E., H. Tosteson, P. M. Ridker, et al. "The Primary Prevention of Myocardial Infarction" *New England Journal of Medicine.* 1992; 326(21):1406–1416.

Taylor, A. E., D. C. Johnson, and H. Kazemi. "AHA Medical/Scientific Statement: Position Statement on Environmental Tobacco Smoke and Cardio-vascular Disease." *Position Paper by the American Heart Association.* 1992.

Willett, W. C., A. Green, M. J. Stamfer, et al. "Relative and Absolute Excess Risks of Coronary Heart Disease Among Women Who Smoke Cigarettes." *New England Journal of Medicine.* 1987; 317:1303–1309.

Chapter 9: Should You Take Estrogen?

Baird, D. T., and A. F. Glasier. "Drug Therapy—Hormonal Contraception." *New England Journal of Medicine.* 1993; 328:1543–1549.

Bar, J., R. Tepper, J. Fuchs, Y. Pardo, S. Goldberger, and J. Ovadia. "The Effect of Estrogen Replacement Therapy on Platelet Aggregation and Adenosine Triphosphate Release in Postmenopausal Women." *Obstetrics and Gynecology.* 1993; 81:261–264.

Barrett-Connor, E. "Estrogen and Coronary Heart Disease in Women." *Journal of the American Medical Association.* 1991; 265:1861–1867.

Bergkvist, L., H.-O. Adami, I. Persson, R. Hoover, and C. Schairer. "The Risk of Breast Cancer After Estrogen and Estrogen-Progestin Replacement." *New England Journal of Medicine.* 1989; 321:293.

Bergkvist, L., H.-O. Adami, I. Persson, R. Bergstrom, and U. B. Krusemo. "Prognosis After Breast Cancer Diagnosis in Women Exposed to Estrogen and Estrogen-Progestogen Replacement Therapy." *American Journal of Epidemiology.* 1989; 130:221.

Bush, T. L., E. Barrett-Connor, L. D. Cowan, M. H. Criqui, R. B. Wallace, C. M. Suchindran, H. A. Tyroler, and B. M. Rifkind. "Cardiovascular Mortality and Noncontraceptive Use of Estrogen in Women: Results from the Lipid Research Clinics Program Follow-up Study." *Circulation.* 1987; 75:1102–1109.

Colditz, G. A., K. M. Egan, and M. J. Stampfer. "Hormone Replacement Therapy and Risk of Breast Cancer: Results from Epidemiologic Studies." *American Journal of Obstetrics and Gynecology.* 1993; 168:1473.

Colditz, G. A., S. E. Hankinson, D. J. Hunter, et al. "The Use of Estrogens and Progestins and the Risk of Breast Cancer in Postmenopausal Women." *New England Journal of Medicine.* 1995; 332:1589–1593.

Colditz, G. A., M. J. Stampfer, W. C. Willett, et al. "Type of Postmenopausal Hormone, Use and Risk of Breast Cancer: 12-Year Follow-up from the Nurses' Health Study." *Cancer Causes and Control.* 1992; 3:433.

Collins, P., G. M. C. Rosano, C. Jiang et al. "Cardiovascular Protection by Oestrogen—A Calcium Antagonist Effect?" *Lancet.* 1993; 341:1264–1265.

Dupont, W. D., and D. L. Page. "Menopausal Estrogen Replacement Therapy and Breast Cancer." *Archives of Internal Medicine.* 1991; 151:67.

Finucane, F. F., J. H. Madans, T. L. Bush, et al. "Decreased Risk of Stroke

Among Postmenopausal Hormone Users." *Archives of Internal Medicine.* 1993; 153:73–79.

Grady, D., S. M. Rubin, D. B. Petitti, et al. "Hormone Therapy to Prevent Disease and Prolong Life in Posmenopausal Women." *Annals of Internal Medicine.* 1992; 117:1016.

Healy, B. "PEPI in Perspective: Good Answers Spawn Pressing Questions." *Journal of the American Medical Association.* 1995; 273:240–242.

Henderson, B. E., A. Paganini-Hill, and R. K. Ross. "Estrogen Replacement Therapy and Protection from Acute Myocardial Infarction." *American Journal of Obstetrics and Gynecology.* 1988; 159:312–317.

Herrstedt, J., T. Sigsgaard, M. Boesgaard, T. P. Jensen, P. Dombernowsky. "Ondansetron Plus Metropimazine Compared with Ondansetron Alone in Patients Receiving Moderately Emetogenic Chemotherapy." *New England Journal of Medicine.* 1993; 328:1076–1080.

Lisbona, H., G. I. Gorodeski, and W. H. Utian. "The Role of Platelets in Prevention of Coronary Heart Disease in Postmenopausal Women—A Review." *Journal of the North American Menopause Society.* 1994; 1(4):227–231.

Martin, K. A., and M. W. Freeman. "Postmenopausal Hormone Replacement Therapy" (Editorial). *New England Journal of Medicine.* 1993; 328:1115–1117.

Nabulsi, A. A., A. R. Folsom, A. White, W. Patsch, G. Heiss, K. K. Wu, and M. Szklo. "Association of Hormone Replacement Therapy with Various Cardiovascular Risk Factors in Postmenopausal Women." *New England Journal of Medicine.* 1993; 328:1069–1075.

Nachtigall, M. J., S. W. Smilen, R. A. D. Nachtigall, R. H. Nachtigall, and L. L. Nachtigall. "Incidence of Breast Cancer in a 22-Year Study of Women Receiving Estrogen-Progestin Replacement Therapy." *Obstetrics and Gynecology.* 1992; 80:827.

Notelovitz, M., S. Katz-Karp, D. Jennings, J. Lancaster, M. Green, and R. W. Stoll. "Effect of Cyclic Estone Sulfate Treatment on Lipid Profiles of Postmenopausal Women with Elevated Cholesterol Levels." *Obstetrics and Gynecology.* 1990; 76:65–70.

Rosano, G. M. C., P. M. Sarrel, P. A. Poole-Wilson, and P. Collins. "Beneficial Effect of Oestrogen on Exercise-induced Myocardial Ischaemia in Women with Coronary Heart Disease." *Lancet.* 1993; 342:133–136.

Sarrel, P. M., E. G. Lufkin, M. J. Oursler, and D. Keefe. "Estrogen Actions in Arteries, Bone and Brain." *Scientific American Science and Medicine.* 1994; 1(3):44–53.

Sarrel, P. M. "Ovarian Hormones and the Circulation." *Maturitas.* 1990; 12:287–298.

Sherwin, B. B., M. M. Gelfand, R. Schucher, et al. "Postmenopausal Estrogen and Androgen Replacement and Lipoprotein Lipid Concentrations." *American Journal of Obstetrics and Gynecology*. 1987; 156:414.

Stampfer, M. J., G. A. Colditz, W. C. Willett, et al. "Postmenopausal Estrogen Therapy and Cardiovascular Disease: Ten-Year Follow-up from the Nurses' Health Study." *New England Journal of Medicine*. 1991; 325:756–762.

Stampfer, M. J., W. C. Willett, G. A. Colditz, F. E. Speizer, and C. H. Hennekens. "A Prospective Study of Past Use of Oral Contraceptive Agents and Risk of Cardiovascular Diseases." *New England Journal of Medicine*. 1988; 319:1313–1317.

Stanford, J. L., N. S. Weiss, L. F. Voigt, et al. "Combined Estrogen and Progestin Hormone Replacement Therapy in Relation to Risk of Breast Cancer in Middle-aged Women." *Journal of the American Medical Association*. 1995; 274:137–142.

Steinberg, K. K., S. B. Thacker, S. J. Smith, D. F. Stroup, M. M. Zach, W. D. Flanders, and R. L. Berkelman. "A Meta-Analysis of the Effect of Estrogen Replacement Therapy on the Risk of Breast Cancer." *Journal of the American Medical Association*. 1991; 265:1985.

Sullivan, J. M., R. VanderZwaag, J. P. Hughes, et al. "Estrogen Replacement and Coronary Artery Disease. Effect on Survival in Postmenopausal Women." *Archives of Internal Medicine*. 1990; 150:2557–2562.

Williams, J. K., D. A. Bellinger, T. C. Nichols, T. R. Griggs, T. F. Bumol, R. L. Fouts, and T. B. Clarkson. "Occlusive Arterial Thrombosis in Cynomolgus Monkeys with Varying Plasma Concentrations of Lipoprotein (a)." *Arteriosclerosis and Thrombosis*. 1993; 13:548–554.

The Writing Group for the PEPI Trial. "Effects of Estrogen or Estrogen/Progestin Regimens on Heart Disease Risk Factors in Postmenopausal Women: The Postmenopausal Estrogen/Progestin Interventional Trial." *Journal of the American Medical Association*. 1995; 273:199–208.

Watts, N. B., M. Notelovitz, M. C. Timmons, et al. "Comparison of Oral Estrogen and Estrogen Plus Androgen on Bone Mineral Density, Menopausal Symptoms, and Lipid and Lipoprotein Profiles in Surgically Menopausal Women." *Obstetrics and Gynecology*. 1995; 85(4):529–537.

Chapter 10: Drugs Used to Prevent Coronary Artery Disease

Havel, R. J., and E. Rapaport. "Drug Therapy—Management of Primary Hyperlipidemia." *New England Journal of Medicine*. 1995; 332:1491–1498.

Levine, G. N., J. F. Keaney, Jr., and J. A. Vita. "Medical Progress—Cholesterol Reduction in Cardiovascular Disease." *New England Journal of Medicine*. 1995; 332:512–521.

Manson, J. E., M. J. Stampfer, G. A. Colditz, et al. "A Prospective Study of

Aspirin Use and Primary Prevention of Cardiovascular Disease in Women." *Journal of the American Medical Association.* 1991; 266:521–527.

Chapter 11: If You Already Have Coronary Artery Disease

Cannon, R. O. "Chest Pain with Normal Coronary Angiograms" (Editorial). *New England Journal of Medicine.* 1993; 328:1706–1708.

Cowley, M. J., S. M. Mullin, S. F. Kelsey, et al. "Sex Differences in Early and Long-term Results of Coronary Angioplasty in the NHLBI PTCA Registry." *Circulation.* 1985; 71:90–97.

Douglas, J. S., S. B. King, E. L. Jones, et al. "Reduced Efficacy of Coronary Artery Bypass Graft Surgery in Women." *Circulation.* 1981: 64(Suppl. 2):11–16.

Egashira, K., T. Inou, Y. Hirooka, A. Yamada, Y. Urabe, and A. Takeshita. "Evidence of Impaired Endothelium-Dependent Coronary Vasodilation in Patients with Angina Pectoris and Normal Coronary Angiograms." *New England Journal of Medicine.* 1993; 328:1659–1664.

James, D. R., Jr., R. Holubkov, R. E. Vliestra, et al. "Comparison of Complications during Percutaneous Transluminal Coronary Angioplasty from 1977 to 1981 and from 1985 to 1986: The National Heart, Lung and Blood Institute Percutaneous Transluminal Coronary Angioplasty Registry." *Journal of the American College of Cardiology.* 1988; 12:1149–1155.

Kane, J. P., M. J. Malloy, T. A. Ports, et al. "Regression of Coronary Atherosclerosis During Treatment of Familial Hypercholesterolemia with Combined Drug Regimens." *Journal of the American Medical Association.* 1990; 264:3007–3012.

McEniery, P. T., J. Hollman, V. Knezinek, et al. "Comparative Safety and Efficacy of Percuntaneous Transluminal Coronary Angioplasty in Men and in Women." *Catheterization and Cardiovascular Diagnosis.* 1987; 13:364–371.

Ornish, D., S. E. Brown, L. W. Scherwitz, et al. "Can Lifestyle Changes Reverse Coronary Heart Disease: The Lifestyle Heart Trial." *Lancet.* 1990; 336:129–133.

Treasure, C. B., J. L. Klein, W. S. Weintraub, et al. "Beneficial Effects of Cholesterol-Lowering Therapy on the Coronary Endothelium in Patients with Coronary Artery Disease." *New England Journal of Medicine.* 1995; 332:481–487.

Chapter 12: If You Have a Heart Attack

Ambrosioni, E., C. Borhi, and B. Magnani. "The Effect of the Angiotensin-Converting-Enzyme Inhibitor Zofenopril on Mortality and Morbidity After

Anterior Myocardial Infarction." *New England Journal of Medicine.* 1995; 332:80–85.

Gallagher, E. J., C. M. Viscoli, and R. I. Horwitz. "The Relationship of Treatment Adherence to the Risk of Death After Myocardial Infarction in Women." *Journal of the American Medical Association.* 1993; 270:742–744.

Pfeffer, M. A. "ACE Inhibition in Acute Myocardial Infarction." *New England Journal of Medicine.* 1995; 332:118–120.

Chapter 13: Hypertension

Black, H. R. "Treatment of Mild Hypertension—The More Things Change . . ." (Editorial). *Journal of the American Medical Association.* 1993; 270:757-759.

The Fifth Report of the Joint National Committee on Detection, Evaluation, and Treatment of High Blood Pressure (JNCV). *Archives of Internal Medicine.* 1993; 153:154–183.

Frolich, E. D., C. Apstein, A. V. Chobanian, et al. "Medical Progress—The Heart in Hypertension." *New England Journal of Medicine.* 1992; 327:998–1008.

Neaton, J. D., R. H. Grimm, Jr., R. J. Prineas, et al. "Treatment of Mild Hypertension Study." *Journal of the American Medical Association.* 1993; 270: 713–724.

Probstfield, J. L. "Prevention of Stroke by Antihypertensive Drug Treatment in Older Persons with Isolated Systolic Hypertension." *Journal of the American Medical Association.* 1991; 265:3255–3264.

Roccella, E. J. "National High Blood Pressure Education Program Working Group Report on Primary Prevention of Hypertension." *ARCH Internal Medicine.* 1993; 154:186–208.

Tjoa, H. I., and N. M. Kaplan. "Treatment of Hypertension in the Elderly." *Journal of the American Medical Association.* 1990; 264:1015–1018.

Victor, R. G., and J. Hansen. "Alcohol and Blood Pressure—A Drink a Day . . ." (Editorial). *New England Journal of Medicine.* 1995; 332:1982–1983.

Winker, M. A., and M. B. Murphy. "Isolated Systolic Hypertension in the Elderly." *Journal of the American Medical Association.* 1991; 265:3301–3302.

Chapter 14: Stroke

Kawachi, I., G. Colditz, M. J. Stampfer, et al. "Smoking Cessation and Decreased Risk of Stroke in Women." *Journal of the American Medical Association.* 1993; 269(2):232–236.

Appendix

Determining Your Body-Mass Index

Turn to the table on pages 284–285. Find your present weight in the left-hand column and read across to the column with your height. If your height or weight doesn't appear on this chart, you can calculate your body-mass index using the following equation:

$$(702.95 \times \text{Weight}) \div (\text{Height} \times \text{Height})$$
$$(\text{in pounds}). \qquad (\text{in inches})$$

For example, if you are 4 feet 11 inches (59 inches) tall and weight 110 pounds, your body-mass index would be

$$(702.95 \times 110) \div (59 \times 59) = 22.21$$

A body-mass index of 27.3 means you are moderately overweight; one of 32.3 indicates severe obesity.

Body-Mass Index Table

Weight (lb):	Height (in): 58	59	60	61	62	63	64	65
110	23.0	22.2	21.5	20.8	20.1	19.5	18.9	18.3
115	24.0	23.2	22.5	21.7	21.0	20.4	19.7	19.1
120	25.1	24.2	23.4	22.7	21.9	21.3	20.6	20.0
125	26.1	25.2	23.4	23.6	22.9	22.1	21.5	20.8
130	27.2	26.3	25.4	24.6	23.8	23.0	22.3	21.6
135	28.2	27.3	26.4	25.5	24.7	23.9	23.2	22.5
140	29.3	28.3	27.3	26.5	25.6	24.8	24.0	23.3
145	30.3	29.3	28.3	27.4	26.5	25.7	24.9	24.1
150	31.4	30.3	29.3	28.3	27.4	26.6	25.7	25.0
155	32.4	31.3	30.3	29.3	28.4	27.5	26.6	25.8
160	33.4	32.3	31.2	30.2	29.3	28.3	27.5	26.6
165	34.5	33.3	32.2	31.2	30.2	29.2	28.3	27.5
170	35.5	34.3	33.2	32.1	31.1	30.1	29.2	28.3
175	36.6	35.3	34.2	33.1	32.0	31.0	30.0	29.1
180	37.6	36.4	35.2	34.0	32.9	31.9	30.9	30.0
185	38.7	37.4	36.1	35.0	33.8	32.8	31.8	30.8
190	39.7	38.4	37.1	35.9	34.8	33.7	32.6	31.6
195	40.8	39.4	38.1	36.8	35.7	34.5	33.5	32.4
200	41.8	40.4	39.1	37.8	36.6	35.4	34.3	33.3
205	42.8	41.4	40.0	38.7	37.5	36.3	35.2	34.1
210	43.9	42.4	41.0	39.7	38.4	37.2	36.0	34.9
215	44.9	43.4	42.0	40.6	39.3	38.1	36.9	35.8
220	46.0	44.4	43.0	41.6	40.2	39.0	37.8	36.6
225	47.0	45.4	43.9	42.5	41.2	39.9	38.6	37.4
230	48.1	46.5	44.9	43.5	42.1	40.7	39.5	38.3
235	49.1	47.5	45.9	44.4	43.0	41.6	40.3	39.1
240	50.2	48.5	46.9	45.3	43.9	42.5	41.2	39.9
245	51.2	49.5	47.8	46.3	44.8	43.4	42.1	40.8
250	52.3	50.5	48.8	47.2	45.7	44.3	42.9	41.6

Body-Mass Index:	Classification:
27.3 to 32.2	Moderate obesity
32.3 and over	Severe obesity

66	67	68	69	70	71	72	73	74
17.8	17.2	16.7	16.2	15.8	15.3	14.9	14.5	14.1
18.6	18.0	17.5	17.0	16.5	16.0	15.6	15.2	14.8
19.4	18.8	18.2	17.7	17.2	16.7	16.3	15.8	15.4
20.2	19.6	19.0	18.5	17.9	17.4	17.0	16.5	16.0
21.0	20.4	19.8	19.2	18.7	18.1	17.6	17.2	16.7
21.8	21.1	20.5	19.9	19.4	18.8	18.3	17.8	17.3
22.6	21.9	21.3	20.7	20.1	19.5	19.0	18.5	18.0
23.4	22.7	22.0	21.4	20.8	20.2	19.7	19.1	18.6
24.2	23.5	22.8	22.2	21.5	20.9	20.3	19.8	19.3
25.0	24.3	23.6	22.9	22.2	21.6	21.0	20.4	19.9
25.8	25.1	24.3	23.6	23.0	22.3	21.7	21.1	20.5
26.6	25.8	25.1	24.4	23.7	23.0	22.4	21.8	21.2
27.4	26.6	25.8	25.1	24.4	23.7	23.1	22.4	21.8
28.2	27.4	26.6	25.8	25.1	24.4	23.7	23.1	22.5
29.1	28.2	27.4	26.6	25.8	25.1	24.4	23.7	23.1
29.9	29.0	28.1	27.3	26.5	25.8	25.1	24.4	23.8
30.7	29.8	28.9	28.1	27.3	26.5	25.8	25.1	24.4
31.5	30.5	29.6	28.8	28.0	27.2	26.4	25.7	25.0
32.3	31.3	30.4	29.5	28.7	27.9	27.1	26.4	25.7
33.1	32.1	31.2	30.3	29.4	28.6	27.8	27.0	26.3
33.9	32.9	31.9	31.0	30.1	29.3	28.5	27.7	27.0
34.7	33.7	32.7	31.8	30.8	30.0	29.2	28.4	27.6
35.5	34.5	33.5	32.5	31.6	30.7	29.8	29.0	28.2
36.3	35.2	34.2	33.2	32.3	31.4	30.5	29.7	28.9
37.1	36.0	35.0	34.0	33.0	32.1	31.2	30.3	29.5
37.9	36.8	35.7	34.7	33.7	32.8	31.9	31.0	30.2
38.7	37.6	36.5	35.4	34.4	33.5	32.6	31.7	30.8
39.5	38.4	37.3	36.2	35.2	34.2	33.2	32.3	31.5
40.4	39.2	38.0	36.9	35.9	34.9	33.9	33.0	32.1

1983 Metropolitan Height and Weight Tables

Although the U.S. Department of Agriculture (USDA) released new weight guidelines in 1990, the guidelines are controversial because they suggest that you can weigh a little more than previously accepted weight standards—particularly in your middle and later years—and still expect good health and a long life. However, recent studies on weight gain and cardiovascular risk in women suggest just the opposite (see page 56). For this reason, we suggest you continue to use the 1983 Metropolitan Life Insurance Company's Height and Weight Tables as a guide for your "ideal" weight.

Remember: the "suggested" weights in all weight tables are just that—a suggestion. The weights in these tables are averages derived from studies of large populations, without regard for individual differences. Hence, you may find that you look fine and feel great at a weight that's higher than those in the weight tables, or you may feel fat at the weight the tables say is right for you. For these reasons, you should work with your physician to determine your ideal weight—the weight that is right for you.

Weights at ages twenty-five through fifty-nine based on lowest mortality. Weight in pounds according to frame (in indoor clothing weighing three pounds for women; shoes with one-inch heels).

WOMEN

| Height | | Small | Medium | Large |
Feet	Inches	Frame	Frame	Frame
4	10	102–111	109–121	118–131
4	11	103–113	111–123	120–134
5	0	104–115	113–126	122–137
5	1	106–118	115–129	125–140
5	2	108–121	118–132	128–143
5	3	111–124	121–135	131–147
5	4	114–127	124–138	134–151
5	5	117–130	127–141	137–155
5	6	120–133	130–144	140–159
5	7	123–136	133–147	143–163
5	8	126–139	136–150	146–167
5	9	129–142	139–153	149–170
5	10	132–145	142–156	152–173
5	11	135–148	145–159	155–176
6	0	138–151	148–162	158–179

Courtesy Metropolitan Life Insurance Company.

Calcium Questionnaire

For each of the following foods you consumed in the last three days, estimate the total amount for each day and write it in columns 1, 2, and 3 (e.g., ½ cup, 6 oz., 5 tbsp., etc.). Then calculate your total calcium intake for the three days by multiplying the amount of calcium in a single serving by the number of servings you had. Add up the total amount of calcium you ate, then divide that number by three. This will give you an estimate of your daily calcium intake. Compare your daily intake with the recommended intakes for women below.

Dairy Products

	Serving Size	Calcium (mg)	1	2	3	Total
MILK Whole	1 cup	288				
Low Fat (2%)	1 cup	352				
Skim & Buttermilk	1 cup	296				
Nonfat, dry	¼ cup	220				
Chocolate	1 cup	278				
Condensed, sweetened	1 cup	802				
Evaporated	1 cup	635				
Lactimilk	1 cup	300				
CHEESE Swiss	1 oz.	262				
Cheddar, Provolone	1 oz.	213				
Edam	1 oz.	207				
Monterey Jack, Mozzarella	1 oz.	200				
Muenster	1 oz.	200				

American, Gouda	1 oz.	198				
Brick	1 oz.	191				
Velveeta (cheese food) 2 tbsp.=	1 oz.	162				
Romano	1 oz.	156				
Blue	1 oz.	150				
Parmesan	1 oz.	136				
Feta	1 oz.	100				
Ricotta (skim)	1 oz.	84				
Ricotta (whole)	1 oz.	65				
Brie	1 oz.	52				
Camembert	1 oz.	30				
Cottage, low fat	1 cup	204				
Cottage, regular	1 cup	131				
OTHER Ice cream (hard)	1 cup	194				
Ice cream (soft)	1 cup	253				
Ice milk (hard)	1 cup	204				
Pudding (instant)	1 cup	374				
Pudding (cooked)	1 cup	265				
Custard (baked)	1 cup	297				
Yogurt, low-fat plain	1 cup	452				
Yogurt, low-fat fruited	1 cup	313				
Yogurt, whole milk	1 cup	275				
Yogurt, frozen	1 cup	220				

Seafood

	Serving Size	Calcium (mg)	1	2	3	Total
Clams, canned (solid/liquid)	1 cup	121				
Mackerel, canned (solid/liquid)	1 cup	552				
Oyster stew (milk, 6 oysters)	1 cup	274				
Salmon, sockeye, canned (solid, liquid w/bones)	1 cup	587				
Sardines, canned (w/bones)	4 med.	69				

Vegetables & Nuts

	Serving Size	Calcium (mg)	1	2	3	Total
Broccoli (frozen, chopped, cooked)	1 cup	100				
Bok choy (chopped, cooked)	1 cup	250				
Collard greens (frozen, chopped, cooked)	1 cup	299				
Kale (frozen, chopped, cooked)	1 cup	157				
Mustard greens (frozen, chopped, cooked)	1 cup	156				
Turnip greens (frozen, chopped, cooked)	1 cup	195				
Beans, all types (dry, cooked, canned, solid/liquid)	1 cup	80				
Almonds (shelled, chopped)	1 cup	304				

Pecans (shelled, chopped)	1 cup	86			
Peanuts (shelled)	1 cup	104			
Mixed nuts, dry roasted peanuts	1 cup	96			
Walnuts, English (shelled, chopped)	1 cup	119			

Miscellaneous

	Serving Size	Calcium (mg)	1	2	3	Total
Tofu	1 oz.	36				
Soybeans (cooked, sprouted)	1 cup	54				
Sunflower seeds (hulled)	1 cup	174				
Cream soups (made with milk)	1 cup	184				
Macaroni and cheese (homemade)	1 cup	362				
Pizza (frozen w/cheese)	4.5" arc	89				
Carob flour	1 cup	480				
Molasses, blackstrap	1 tbsp.	137				

Calcium-Fortified Foods

	Serving Size	Calcium (mg)	1	2	3	Total
Minute Maid orange juice	1 cup	320				
Calci-Milk	1 cup	500				

Total Calcium _____

Average Daily Calcium Intake _____
  (Divide Total Calcium by 3)

RECOMMENDED CALCIUM INTAKE FOR WOMEN

Age	Optimal Daily Intake
Children ages 1–10 years old	800
Teenagers	1,200–1,500
Women:	
Ages 25 to 50	
• Premenopausal	1,000
• Surgical or premature natural menopause	1,500
Over 50	
• Not taking estrogen	1,500
• Taking estrogen	1,000
Pregnant or nursing	Additional 400

Fitness Norms for Women

Resting Heart Rate (beats per minute)

Norm	18–25	26–35	36–45	46–55	56–65	Over 65
Excellent	54–60	54–59	54–59	54–60	54–59	54–59
Good	61–65	60–64	62–64	61–65	61–64	60–64
Above Average	66–69	66–68	66–69	66–69	67–69	66–68
Average	70–73	69–71	70–72	70–73	71–73	70–72
Below Average	74–78	72–76	74–78	74–77	75–77	73–76
Poor	80–84	78–82	79–82	78–84	79–81	79–84
Very Poor	86–100	84–94	84–92	85–96	85–96	88–96

Column group heading: AGE

Fitness norms for resting heart rate reprinted from *Y's Ways to Physical Fitness*, 3rd ed. (Champaign, IL: Human Kinetics Publishers, 1989), with permission of the YMCA of the USA, 101 N. Wacker Drive, Chicago, IL 60606.

Maximal Oxygen Uptake (VO$_2$max) (ml/kg min)

Norm	18–25	26–35	36–45	46–55	56–65	Over 65
Excellent	58–71	54–69	46–66	42–64	38–57	33–51
Good	48–54	46–51	39–44	35–39	32–36	28–31
Above Average	42–46	40–43	34–37	31–33	28–31	25–27
Average	39–41	35–38	31–33	28–30	25–27	22–24
Below Average	34–37	31–34	28–30	25–27	22–24	20–22
Poor	29–32	26–30	23–26	21–24	19–21	17–18
Very Poor	18–26	20–25	18–21	16–19	14–17	14–16

Column group heading: AGE

Fitness Norms for maximal oxygen uptake reprinted from *Y's Ways to Physical Fitness*, 3rd ed. (Champaign, IL: Human Kinetics Publishers, 1989), with permission of the YMCA of the USA, 101 N. Wacker Drive, Chicago, IL 60606.

YOUR PERSONAL FITNESS PROFILE

	Baseline	3 weeks	6 weeks	3 months	6 months
Weight					
Resting Heart Rate					
Maximal Oxygen Uptake (VO$_2$max) or One-Mile Walk					

Walking Field Test

The tables here are to be used in conjunction with the walking field test (described on page 122). To take the test, first, walk one mile (on a flat surface) as fast as you can. This should take you anywhere between ten and twenty-five minutes. Record your time to the nearest second. *Immediately* take your pulse after you have completed the walk.

To see how your performance compares with other women your age, find the relative fitness graph for your age group. On the scale along the bottom of the graph, mark the time it took you to walk one mile. (Be sure to choose the time scale that corresponds with your weight, as indicated on the right side of the scale.) On the left side of the scale, mark your heart rate at the end of the walk. Now draw a vertical line from your walk time and a horizontal line from your heart rate to the point where they intersect. The area where these two points meet shows your relative fitness level for your age and weight: either high, above average, average, below average, or low. Create your own "Personal Fitness Profile," opposite page, to chart your progress.

Fitness Norms for Women: Walking Field

Relative Fitness Level Chart for 20- to 29-Year-Old Females

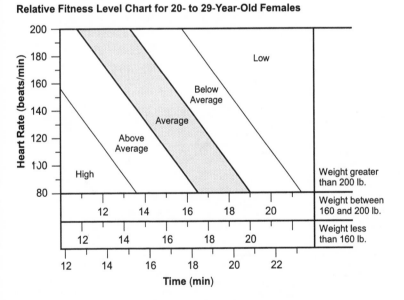

Note: Fitness norms for the Walking Field Test based on the One Mile Walk Test developed by Dr. James Rippe and colleagues. Reprinted from *The Rockport Walking Program* (New York: Prentice Hall, 1989), with permission of the author.

Relative Fitness Level Chart for 30- to 39-Year-Old Females

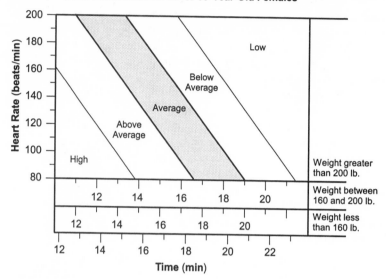

Relative Fitness Level Chart for 40- to 49-Year-Old Females

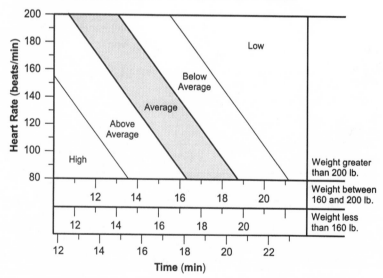

Relative Fitness Level Chart for 50- to 59-Year-Old Females

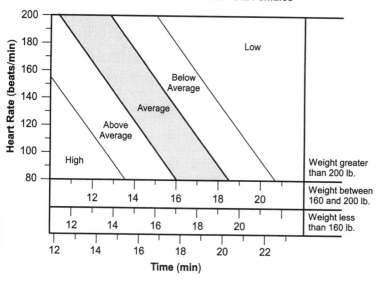

Relative Fitness Level Chart for 60- to 69-Year-Old Females

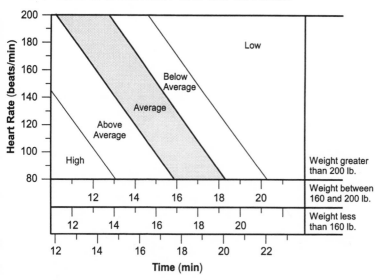

Index

Adolescents, cholesterol tests for, 68–69

Adrenergic inhibitors, 221

Aerobic vs. nonaerobic activities, 119–120

Age
risk of coronary artery disease and, 2–4, 48–49
risk of hypertension and, 213
risk of stroke and, 227–228

Alcohol consumption, 138–139
hypertension and, 214, 218
risk of stroke and, 231, 234–235

American Diabetes Association, 257

American Dietetic Association, 83, 257–258

American Heart Association, 256
smoking statistics of, 51–52
Step I diet, 200

American Lung Association, 259–260

Americans vs. French, eating habits of, 110–112

Anatomy and physiology
cardiovascular system, 13–24
female vs. male, 25–30

Anderson, Dr. James W., 177

Androgen therapy, 166–167

Anger, suppression of and heart disease, 59, 145

Angina
definition of, 20
microvascular, 185
See also Chest pain

Angioplasty, 193–195, 206

Angiotensin-converting enzyme (ACE) inhibitors, 207, 221

Ankle/Arm Blood Pressure Index (AAI), 66

Antiarrhythmics, 184, 206–207

Anticoagulants, 179–180, 185, 207, 238, 240

Antioxidants, 100–102

Antiplatelet drugs, 178–179, 185, 207, 238

Antithrombic drugs, 178–180, 238, 240

Anxiety, 145. *See also* Stress

Apolipoproteins, 37–38

Arrhythmias, 23–24, 205, 243–249, 252–253

Arteriosclerosis, definition of, 18, 48–49. *See also* Cholesterol

Artery spasms, reduction of blood flow by, 44

Artery wall, atherosclerosis and, 41–42

Aspirin, 178–179, 185, 207, 231–232, 235

Asymptomatic carotid bruit, 229–230

Atherosclerosis
  antioxidants and, 100–102
  definition of, 18–20
  development of, 33–47
  See also Coronary artery disease

Atrial fibrillation, 246–247

B vitamins, 63, 106–107

Bacterial endocarditis, 249–250, 253–254

Baldness, risk of coronary artery disease and, 62

Balloon angioplasty, 193–195, 206

Beta-blockers, 182, 207, 220–221

Bicycle test, 123

Bicycling program (beginner's), 127

Bile acid sequestrants, 176

Biphasic oral contraceptives, 153

Birth control pills, 5, 26, 147–155
  blood clots and, 45
  congenital heart defects and, 253–254
  risk of stroke and, 232–233
  risk of hypertension and, 214

Blair, Steven, 117

Blood clots
  antithrombic drugs, 178–180
  birth control pills and, 148
  development of coronary heart disease and, 37–38
  estrogen and, 45–46, 156, 169
  exercise as prevention for, 118
  physiology of, 16–18
  thrombolytic therapy for heart attack, 205–206
  See also Stroke

Blood homocysteine levels, 72

Blood pressure
  classifications for, 216
  estrogen's effect on, 44–45
  physiology of, 15–16
  risk of coronary artery disease and, 51

  screening for coronary artery disease and, 66
  See also Hypertension; Hypotension

Blood vessels, physiology of, 15

Body fat, measuring, 64–65

Body-mass index (BMI), 65, 283–285

Bone mass, birth control pills and, 150

Bradycardia, 23, 248

Breast cancer
  birth control pills and, 151
  estrogen therapy and, 160–162
  myth about, 2

Bypass surgery, 30, 196–199, 206

Caffeine, 106, 109

Calcium, 104–106
  hypertension and, 219
  questionnaire, 287–290
  recommended intake, 291

Calcium channel blockers, 184, 221

Cancer
  birth control pills and, 150–151
  estrogen therapy and, 159–163, 167
  myth about, 2

Carbohydrates, complex, 96–98

Cardiac catheterization, 77–78

Cardiac medications, 181–192

Cardiovascular conditions, 243–254

Cardiovascular system, description of, 13–24
  anatomy of, 13–18
  cardiovascular conditions, 24
  coronary artery disease, 18–22

Carotid
  bruit, 229–230
  endarterectomy, 238–239
  pulse, taking, 126

Central alpha agonists, 222

Cerebral embolism, 227. *See also* Stroke

Cerebral hemorrhage, 227. *See also* Stroke

Cerebral thrombosis, 226–227. *See also* Stroke

Chest pain
  attending to, 21, 203–204

diagnosing, 76–77
myth about, 4
See also Angina
Children
    atherosclerosis in, 47
    cholesterol tests for, 68–69
Cholesterol
    age and levels of, 27
    antioxidants and, 100–102
    birth control pills and, 147–148
    blood clot development and, 38
    development of coronary heart
        disease and, 34–37
    diet and, 86
    dietary fiber and, 96–98
    estrogen and, 25–26, 28, 44, 156,
        159, 169, 173
    exercise and, 118, 120
    lipid-lowering drugs, 175–178
    myth about, 5–6
    risk of stroke and, 234
    risk of coronary artery disease and,
        49–51
    screening for coronary artery
        disease and, 5–6, 67–71
    See also Atherosclerosis
Cholesterol-Saturated Fat Index
    (CSI), 94–95
Cigarette smoking, 51–52, 133–138
    birth control pills and, 152, 154
    estrogen therapy and, 167, 169
    resources for support to quit,
        259–260
    risk of stroke and, 231, 234
Circadian rhythms, 130
Clarkson, Dr. Thomas B., 47
Clots. *See* Blood clots
Cocaine abuse, risk of coronary artery
    disease and, 62
Coffee, 106, 109
Colon cancer, estrogen and, 162–163
Congenital heart defects, 252–254
Connor, Sonja L. and William E., 94
Contraceptives, oral, 5, 26, 147–155
    blood clots and, 45
    congenital heart defects and,
        253–254
    risk of hypertension and, 214
    risk of stroke and, 232–233

Coronary angioplasty, 193–195, 206
Coronary artery bypass graft surgery
    (CAGB), 30, 196–199, 206
Coronary artery disease
    development of, 33–47
    diet to prevent, 80–116
    drugs to prevent, 175–180
    estrogen therapy and, 146–174
    exercise to prevent, 117–132
    heart attack patients, 202–208
    myths about, 1–9
    overview of, 18–22
    resources and support, 256–257
    risk factors for, 48–63, 133–145
    screening and diagnostic tests for,
        64–79
    therapy for, 181–201
Coronary Artery Surgery Study
    (CASS), 30
Cyanosis, 253

Decaffeinated coffee, 109
Depression, 145
Diabetes
    coronary risk factors of, 55–56,
        140–142, 230, 234
    development of coronary heart
        disease and, 38–39
    estrogen therapy and, 169
    exercise and, 118
    fasting blood glucose test, 70–71
    resources and support, 257
Diagnostic tests for coronary artery
    disease, 72–79
Diet
    diabetes and, 141
    prevention of coronary artery
        disease and, 80–116
    stress and, 142
Diuretics, 220
Drug abuse, 29, 231, 259–260. *See
    also* Alcohol consumption
Drugs
    antithrombics, 178–180, 238, 240
    cardiac medications, 181–192
    heart attack, emergency treatment
        of, 205–207
    hypertensive medications,
        220–222

Drugs (*Cont.*)
  lipid-lowering, 175–178
  prevention of coronary artery
    disease, 175–180
  stroke treatment, 238, 240
  See also Estrogen; Oral
    contraceptives

Eating, time of day and, 110–112. *See
  also* Diet
Echocardiogram, 76
Eisenmenger's Syndrome, 254
Electrocardiogram (ECG), 72–73
Ellison, Dr. R. Curtis, 110–111
Emotional stress
  exercise and, 118
  hypertension and, 214–215,
    219–220
  risk factor of, 142–145
  risk of coronary artery disease and,
    58–60
Endocarditis, bacterial, 249–250,
  253–254
Endometrial cancer
  birth control pills and, 150
  estrogen therapy and, 158–160
Estrogen, 146–174
  combination therapy with
    progestogen, 163–166
  development of coronary heart
    disease and, 42–47
  dietary, 102–104
  hypertension and, 221–222
  myth about, 5
  postmenopausal therapy,
    155–174, 184–185
  protective power of, 25–28
  stroke and, 232–233
  See also Oral contraceptives
Ethic background, risk of coronary
  artery disease and, 57–58, 229
Exercise
  diabetes and, 141
  hypertension and, 217
  minimizing risks of, 128–131
  prevention of coronary artery
    disease and, 117–132
  program for women with heart
    disease, 127–128

risk of coronary artery disease and,
  52
risk of stroke and, 235
stress and, 142
See also Fitness
Exercise stress test, 73–74, 122–123

Familial defective Apo B-100, 53
Familial hypercholesterolemia, 37,
  52, 200
Familial hypertriglyceridemia, 35
Fasting blood glucose test, 70–71
Fats, dietary, 83–95
  calories, counting, 89–90
  cutting back on, 90–95
  grams, counting, 88–89
  types of, 84–87
Fatty acids, 84
FDA (Food and Drug
  Administration), 258
Female anatomy and physiology,
  25–30
Fiber, dietary, 96–100, 105–106
Fibric acids, 177
Fibrinogen, estrogen and, 45–46, 62,
  158
Fibrocystic breast disease, 150
Fitness
  evaluating levels of, 122–125
  norms for women, 291–295
  See also Exercise
Flavonoids, 102, 109
Follicle stimulating hormone (FSH),
  55
Food and Nutrition Information
  Center, 258
Framingham Heart Study, 7
  angina statistics, 20
  heart attack statistics, 22
  homocysteine levels, 63
  hysterectomy and risk of heart
    disease, 55
  pregnancy and heart disease, 27
  triglyceride levels and heart
    disease, 35
  working women and heart disease.
    59
Free radicals, 36
  antioxidants, 100–102

iron storage and, 60
French vs. Americans, eating habits
    of, 110–112

Gallstones, estrogen and, 163
Gender
    dietary recommendations and,
        81–82
    heart disease and, 2–3, 25–30, 49
    medical care and, 6–7
    risk of stroke and, 228
Genetics
    risk of coronary artery disease and,
        52–54
    risk of hypertension and, 213
    risk of stroke and, 229
Glucose tolerance test, 71
Graded exercise stress test, 122–123

Heart
    anatomy of, 13–24
    beating of, 243–244
    conduction system of, 245
    congenital defects of, 252–254
    See also Cardiovascular conditions;
        Coronary artery disease;
        Hypertension; Stroke
Heart attack
    definition of, 22
    patient lifestyles, 202–208
    warning signs of, 21
Heart block, 248–249
Heart valves, problems with,
    249–252
Heat shock proteins, 41
Heredity
    risk of coronary artery disease and,
        52–54
    risk of hypertension and, 213
    risk of stroke and, 229
High blood pressure. See
    Hypertension
High-density lipoproteins (HLD),
    36–37. See also Cholesterol
Holter monitor, 77
Homocysteine levels, 63
    blood test for, 72
    diet and, 106–107

Hormone replacement therapy. See
    Estrogen
Hypertension, 211–225
    birth control pills and, 148–149
    calcium and, 104–106
    definition of, 22–23, 211–212
    diagnosing, 215–216
    estrogen and, 156, 168
    exercise and, 117–118
    insulin and, 39
    lifestyle for lowering, 216–220
    medications for, 220–222
    risks of, 51, 139, 213–215, 230,
        234
    screening for coronary artery
        disease and, 66
    sodium and, 98
Hypotension, 182, 184, 222–225
Hysterectomy, risk of coronary artery
    disease and, 54–55

Immune system, development of
    coronary heart disease and,
        39–41
Infective endocarditis, 249–250, 253
Insulin
    birth control pills and, 148
    development of coronary heart
        disease and, 38–39
    estrogen and, 46, 156
    exercise and, 118
    fasting blood glucose test, 70–71
    See also Diabetes
Iron, 60–61, 107
Iron-deficiency anemia, birth control
    pills and, 151
Ischemia, silent, 20
Isoflavones, 103–104

Kidneys, blood pressure and, 15–16

Left ventricular hypertrophy, 76
Lerner, Harriet Goldhor, 145
Lifestyle
    blood pressure lowering tips,
        216–220
    coronary artery disease patients,
        199–201
Lifestyle evaluation, 79

Lindsay, Dr. Robert, 150
Lipid profile. See Cholesterol, screening
Lipoproteins. See Cholesterol
Low blood pressure, 182, 184, 222–225
Low-density lipoproteins (LDL), 36. See also Cholesterol

Macrophages, 39–40
Manson, Dr. JoAnn, 56
Mast cells, 40
Maximal exercise stress test, 122–123
Maximal oxygen consumption (VO₂max), 122, 292
Maximum heart rate and target zone, determining, 124–125
Medications. See Drugs
Melanoma, estrogen therapy and, 167
Menopause
    heart disease statistics and, 28
    risk of coronary artery disease and, 54
    See also Estrogen
Metropolitan Life Height and Weight Tables, 286
Microvascular angina, 20, 185
Mitral valve prolapse (MVP), 24, 249–252
Modified GXT, 123
Monocytes, 39–40
Monophasic oral contraceptives, 152–153
Monounsaturated fats, 85, 87
Myocardial infarction. See Heart attack
Myths about coronary artery disease, 1–9

National Clearinghouse for Alcohol and Drug Abuse Information, 259
National Diabetes Information Clearinghouse, 257
National Heart, Lung and Blood Institute, 30, 256–257
National Health and Nutrition Examination Survey, 27

National Menopause Foundation, 260
Niacin, cholesterol-lowering usage of, 176
NIH Panel on Triglycerides and HDL Cholesterol, 49–51, 81
Nitrates (nitroglycerine), 182–183, 207
Nurses' Health Study, 179
Nutritional evaluation, 82–83
Nuts, 107–108

Oat bran, cholesterol and, 96–97
Obesity. See Weight
Omega-3 fatty acids, 85
Oral contraceptives, 5, 26, 147–155
    blood clots and, 45
    congenital heart defects and, 253–254
    risk of hypertension and, 214
    risk of stroke and, 232–233
Ornish, Dr. Dean, 82, 93, 200
Orthostatic hypotension, 182, 184, 222–225
Ovarian cancer
    birth control pills and, 150
    estrogen therapy and, 162–163
Ovariectomy, risk of coronary artery disease and, 54–55
Overeaters Anonymous, 259

Paroxysmal atrial tachycardia, 246
Pathobiological Determinants of Atherosclerosis in Youth (PDAY) study, 47
Pattern baldness, risk of coronary artery disease and, 62
Pelvic inflammatory disease, birth control pills and, 151
Percutaneous transluminal coronary angioplasty (PTCA), 193–195, 206
Peripheral arterial disease (PAD), 66
Physical fitness
    evaluating levels of, 122–125
    norms for women, 291–295
    See also Exercise
Physiology
    cardiovascular system, 13–24

female vs. male, 25–30
Phytoestrogens, 102–104
Plaque, formation of, 43. *See also* Cholesterol
Polycythemia, 253
Polyunsaturated fats, 85, 87
Postmenopausal Estrogen-Progestin Interventions (PEPI) Trial, 44–45, 155, 157–159
Postmenopausal hormone preparations, 170–172. *See also* Estrogen
Potassium, hypertension and, 219
PPP Principle, 112
Pregnancy
  congenital heart defects and, 254
  heart disease and, 26–27
  -induced hypertension, 214
Premature atrial contractions, 247–248
Premature beats, 23
Premature ventricular contractions, 247–248
Probucol, 100–101, 177
Progestogen
  oral contraceptives, 153, 155
  therapy, 163–166, 173
Psyllium seed, cholesterol and, 97–98, 177–178
Pulse, taking, 126

Radial pulse, taking, 126
Red blood cell count, 230
Relative Fitness Level Charts, 293–295
Relaxation techniques, 142–143. *See also* Stress
Resistance weight training, 119–120
Resources and support, 256–260
Resting electrocardiogram (ECG), 72–73
Resting heart rate, 125, 292
Rheumatic heart disease, 24
Risk factors, coronary artery disease, 48–63, 133–145

Salt, blood pressure and, 16, 98, 106, 213, 218
Saturated fats, 84–85, 87. *See also*

Cholesterol-Saturated Fat Index (CSI)
Screening tests for coronary artery disease, 64–72
Silent ischemia, definition of, 20
Silent myocardial infarction, 22
Sinoatrial node, 245
Sinus tachycardia, 246
Skin cancer, estrogen therapy and, 167
Skin-fold test, 65
Sleep, stress and, 143
Smoking, 51–52, 133–138
  birth control pills and, 152, 154
  estrogen therapy and, 167, 169
  resources for support to quit, 259–260
  risk of stroke and, 231, 234
Social role of women, cardiovascular disease and, 28–30
Sodium, 16, 98, 106, 213, 218
Soy proteins, 103–104
Stampfer, Dr. Meir, 138, 149
Statins, 176–177
Stationary bicycling program (beginner's), 127
Stress
  exercise and, 118
  hypertension and, 214–215, 219–220
  relieving, 143
  risk factors of, 58–60, 142–145
Stress test, 73–74, 122–123
Stroke, 23, 226–242
  antithrombic drugs for, 178–180, 238, 240
  estrogen therapy and, 155
  preventing, 233–235
  risk factors for, 227–233
  treatment for, 235–242
  types of, 228
Stroke Connection Network, 242
Subarachnoid hemorrhage, 227
Substance abuse, 29, 231, 259–260. *See also* Alcohol consumption
Superko, Dr. Robert, 111
Supplements, 109–110

Syndrome X
  angina, 21
  diabetic cholesterol levels, 38

Tachycardia, 23, 245–246
Taking Off Pounds Sensibly (TOPS)
  Club, 258–259
Target heart range, determining,
  124–125
Tea, 102, 109
Teenagers, cholesterol tests for,
  68–69
Testosterone, cholesterol levels and,
  26
Tests, screening and diagnostic for
  coronary artery disease,
  64–79
Thallium exercise stress test, 74–75
Thiazide diuretics, 220
Thrombolytic therapy, 205–206
Thrombosis. *See* Blood clots
Time of day
  eating and, 110–112
  exercise and, 130–131
Tobacco. *See* Smoking
Trans fatty acids, 86, 87
Transient ischemic attacks (TIAs),
  230–231, 235
Triglyceride bulge, 111–112
Triglycerides, 35, 50–51, 81, 84
Triglyceride-tolerance test, 72
Triphasic oral contraceptives, 153
Tubal ligation, 254
Type III hyperlipoproteinemia, 53
Type A personality, 28, 59

Unstable angina, 20
Uric acid test, 71

Vasodilators, 221

Vegetarian diet, 93–94
Ventricular fibrillation, 248
Very-low-density lipoproteins
  (VLDL), 35–36. *See also*
  Cholesterol
Virmani, Dr. Renu, 62
Vitamin
  antioxidants, 100–102
  B, 63, 106–107
  supplements, 109–110

Waist-to-hip ratio, 65
Walking program (beginner's),
  125–127
Walking field test, 123–124, 293
Weight
  Body-Mass Index Table, 283–
  285
  diabetes and, 141–142
  hypertension and, 213, 217
  Metropolitan Life Height and
  Weight Tables, 286
  quitting smoking and, 136–137
  resources and support to control,
  257–259
  risk factors of, 56–57, 139–140,
  231, 235
  screening for coronary artery
  disease and, 64–65
  tips for loss of, 113–114
Weight Watchers International, 259
Willett, Dr. Walter C., 56–57, 86
Wine, consumption of, 111–112
Women to Woman America, 260
Women vs. men
  dietary recommendations for,
  81–82
  heart disease and, 2–3
  medical care and, 6–7
  physiological differences, 25–30

Permissions Acknowledgments

Death Rates from Coronary Heart Disease: A Comparison of Men and Women, on page 3, reprinted from Bush, T.L., "The Epidemiology of Cardiovascular Disease in Postmenopausal Women," in *Annals of the New York Academy of Sciences,* vol. 592, page 265,1990 with permission from the publisher and the author.

Levels of HDL and LDL Cholesterol Throughout a Woman's Lifetime, on page 27, reprinted from Knopp, R.H., J.C. LaRosa, and R.T. Burkman Jr., "Contraception and Dyslipidemia," in *The American Journal of Obstetrics and Gynecology,* vol. 168, pages 1994–2005, 1993 with permission from the publisher.

Cholesterol Levels and Heart Disease Risk, on page 50, reprinted from Martin, M., W. Browner, S. Hulley, L. Kuller, and D. Wentworth, "Serum Cholesterol, Blood Pressure, and Mortality: Implications from a Cohort of 361,622 Men" in *The Lancet,* October 25, 1986 with permission from the publisher.

The Cholesterol-Saturated Fat Index of Some Common Foods, on page 95, reprinted from Connor, S.L., et al., "The Cholesterol Saturated Fat Index: An Indication of the Hypercholestroaemic and Atherogenic Potential of Food," in *The Lancet,* May 31, 1986, with permission from the publisher.

High-Fiber Foods, on pages 99–100, excerpted from Anderson, J.W., *Plant Fiber in Foods* (Lexington, KY: HCF Nutrition Research Foundation, Inc., 1990). Copyright © 1990 by James W. Anderson, M.D.

The Triglyceride Bulge, on page 112, reprinted from Cohn, J.S., J.R. McNamara and E.J. Schaefer, "Lipoprotein Cholesterol Concentrations in the Plasma of Human Subjects as Measured in the Fed and Fasted States," in *Clinical Chemistry,* vol. 34, no. 10, pages 2456–2459, 1989, with permission from the publisher.

Relative Risk of Heart Attacks Among Smoking and Non-smoking Users of Oral Contraceptives on page 154 adapted from Croft, P., and P.C. Hannaford, "Risk Factors for Acute Myocardial Infarction in Women: Evidence from the Royal College of General Practitioners' Oral Contraception Study," in *British Medical Journal,* vol. 298, pages 165–168, 1989, with permission from the publisher and the authors.

Breast Cancer Risk Associated with Estrogen Use, on page 161, reprinted from Dupont, W., and D.L. Page, "Menopausal Estrogen Replacement Therapy and Breast Cancer," in *Archives of Internal Medicine,* vol. 151, no. 1, pages 67–72, 1991.

The 1983 Metropolitan Height and Weight Tables on page 286, reprinted with permission from the Metropolitan Life Insurance Company.

Fitness Norms for Maximal Oxygen Uptake and Resting Heart Rate (page 292), reprinted from *Y's Ways to Physical Fitness, 3rd ed.* (Champaign, IL: Human Kinetics Publishers, 1989), with permission of the YMCA of the USA, 101 N. Wacker Drive, Chicago, IL 60606.

Fitness Norms for the Walking Field Test that appear on page 293–295 are based on the One Mile Walk Test developed by Dr. James Rippe and colleagues. Reprinted from *The Rockport Walking Program* (New York, NY: Prentice Hall Publishers, 1989), with permission of the author.

ABOUT THE AUTHORS

Morris Notelovitz, M.D., Ph.D., was the founder of the Center for Climacteric Studies at the University of Florida and is currently the president of The Women's Medical & Diagnostic Center, the nation's first facilities to integrate both research and treatment for adult women. He has supervised research on women, and has been an outspoken proponent for their rights and obligations as health-care consumers. A pioneer in the field of women's health, he was among the first to bring national attention to osteoporosis, its treatment, risk factors, and preventive care, in the book *Stand Tall! The Informed Women's Guide to Preventing Osteoporosis* (written with Marsha Ware and Diana Tonnessen), and he was instrumental in pioneering women's birth-room options that are now the mainstay for births in hospitals around the country.

Dr. Notelovitz has had a specialized interest in menopause and midlife health issues for twenty-five years, and was an early advocate of menopause management rather than symptom-oriented treatment. Past chairman of the International Menopause Society, he is founder and president of The National Menopause Foundation, Inc., an organization that advocates research on menopause and that administers 800 and 900 numbers (1-800-MENOASK; 1-900-678-MENO), which answer women's questions about menopause and other midlife health issues. The foundation also supports the Women to Woman America program, whose mission is to help women in their midlife years achieve a healthy body in a healthy environment. A NOVA program, "What's New About Menopause," featured The Women's

Medical and Diagnostic Center and Climacteric Clinic as a model facility where women can receive integrated care.

Dr. Notelovitz is also the publisher of *Women's Health Digest*, a medical journal written by experts for the consumer. With Diana Tonnessen, he has written several books on women's health care and related issues, including *Stand Tall! The Informed Women's Guide to Preventing Osteoporosis* (with Marsha Ware), *Menopause & Midlife Health,* and *Estrogen: Yes or No?*

Diana Tonnessen has more than ten years of experience as a medical reporter, feature writer, magazine editor, and book author. She is the author of *50 Essential Things to Do When the Doctor Says It's Diabetes,* and coauthor of seven other books. Her magazine articles have appeared in *McCall's, Glamour, Self, Working Mother,* and *Health.* She lives in Reston, Virginia.